Optical Coherence Tomography - Developments and Innovations in Ophthalmology

Edited by Giuseppe Lo Giudice and Irene Gattazzo

Published in London, United Kingdom

Optical Coherence Tomography - Developments and Innovations in Ophthalmology
http://dx.doi.org/10.5772/intechopen.98051
Edited by Giuseppe Lo Giudice and Irene Gattazzo

Contributors
Svetlana Zhukova, Tatiana Iureva, Dmitry Samsonov, Karanjit Kooner, Sruthi Suresh, Emily Buchanan, Hafsa Zuberi, Mohannad Albdour, Mahad Rehman, Mobin Ibne Mokbul, Sherin Sadek, Ragai Hatata, Luis Niño-de-Rivera, Erwin-Michel Davila-Iniesta, Amin Zand, Alessandro Arrigo, Francesco Bandello, Lorenzo Bianco, Alessio Antropoli, Andrea Saladino, Alessandro Berni, Maurizio Battaglia Parodi, Artemiy Kokhanov, Ye He, Pooja Nikki Bisarya, Irena Tsui, Sumathi Manickam, I. Rexiline Sheeba, K. Venkatraman

First published in London, United Kingdom, 2023 by IntechOpen
IntechOpen is the global imprint of INTECHOPEN LIMITED, registered in England and Wales, registration number: 11086078, 5 Princes Gate Court, London, SW7 2QJ, United Kingdom

British Library Cataloguing-in-Publication Data
A catalogue record for this book is available from the British Library

Additional hard and PDF copies can be obtained from orders@intechopen.com

Optical Coherence Tomography - Developments and Innovations in Ophthalmology
Edited by Giuseppe Lo Giudice and Irene Gattazzo
p. cm.
Print ISBN 978-1-80355-072-5
Online ISBN 978-1-80355-073-2
eBook (PDF) ISBN 978-1-80355-074-9

Meet the editors

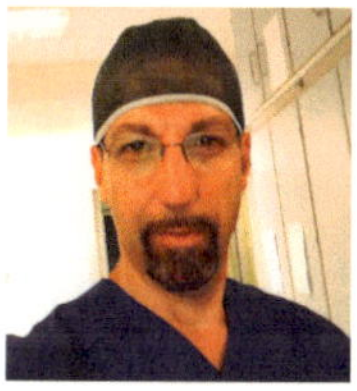

Giuseppe Lo Giudice obtained an MD from the University of Messina, Italy. He completed his ophthalmological residency at the Department of Ophthalmology, University of Padua, Italy, after residency training. He was a fellow in the Ophthalmology Department of the Gironcoli Ophthalmic Center from 2002 to 2004. He was an assistant in ophthalmology at Conegliano Hospital Conegliano, Treviso, Italy from 2004 to 2007. Since 2007, Dr. Lo Giudice has been a surgeon and vice-director at San Antonio Hospital, University of Padua. His major fields of interest are treatments for retinal diseases (proliferative retinopathies, age-related macular degeneration, and diabetic retinopathy) and vitreoretinal surgery. He has more than 25 years of experience in clinical research as well as in clinical trials and laboratory research. He performed more than 9000 anterior segment surgeries (cataract surgery, glaucoma surgery, corneal transplantation) in the last 5 years and more than 2000 vitreo-retinal surgeries for several vitreoretinal diseases (ocular trauma, complicated cataract surgery, retinal pucker, retinal detachment, and vitreoretinal proliferative disease) in the last 3 years.

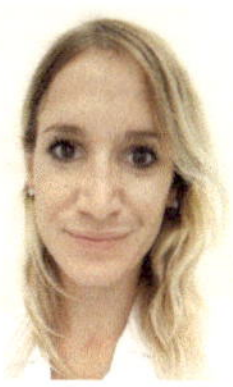

Irene Gattazzo graduated in Medicine and Surgery from the University of Padua, Italy, in 2016. She then specialized in ophthalmology at the Sapienza University of Rome, Italy, in 2022. During her training, she showed interest in different fields of ophthalmology and participated in several research projects, with a predilection for retinal imaging.

Contents

Preface **IX**

Section 1
Optical Coherence Tomography and Retina **1**

Chapter 1 **3**
Role of OCT Angiography OCTA in the Diagnosis of Macular Diseases
by Sherin Sadek and Ragai Hatata

Chapter 2 **17**
OCT from the Past to the Future
by Sherin Sadek and Ragai Hatata

Chapter 3 **27**
New OCT and OCTA Insights in Inherited Retinal Dystrophies
by Alessandro Arrigo, Lorenzo Bianco, Alessio Antropoli, Andrea Saladino, Alessandro Berni, Maurizio Battaglia Parodi and Francesco Bandello

Chapter 4 **49**
Optical Coherence Tomography in Retinopathy of Prematurity
by Artemiy Kokhanov, Ye He, Pooja Nikki Bisarya and Irena Tsui

Section 2
Optical Coherence Tomography and Optic Nerve **65**

Chapter 5 **67**
The Role of Optical Coherence Tomography Angiography in Glaucoma
by Karanjit Kooner, Mahad Rehman, Sruthi Suresh, Emily Buchanan, Mohannad Albdour and Hafsa Zuberi

Chapter 6 **91**
Morphofunctional Changes of the Retina and Optic Nerve in Optical Neuropathy of Various Genesis: A Literature Review
by Svetlana Zhukova, Tatiana Iureva and Dmitry Samsonov

Chapter 7 **111**
Optic Neuropathies
by Amin Zand

Chapter 8 129
Optical Coherence Tomography Angiography (OCT-A): Emerging Landscapes in Neuro-Ophthalmology and Central Nervous System (CNS) Disorders
by Mobin Ibne Mokbul

Section 3
Optical Coherence Tomography and Miscellaneous 151

Chapter 9 153
Study and Analysis of Fluid Filled Abnormalities in Retina Using OCT Images
by Sumathi Manickam, I. Rexiline Sheeba and K. Venkatraman

Chapter 10 163
A New Method to Manipulate Conventional OCT Images to Measure Changes in the Relative Haemoglobin Oxygen Saturation
by Erwin-Michel Davila-Iniesta and Luis Niño-de-Rivera

Preface

One may ask why we need another book about optical coherence tomography (OCT). It's a fair question and I agree that there is already an abundance of literature on this topic. However, we must also consider that OCT has totally changed the paradigm of ophthalmology since its first appearance. The progress made in ophthalmic imaging technologies in the past two decades has changed both clinical and diagnostic approaches in ocular diseases while also improving the efficiency of eye care. The ability to visualize ocular structures in vivo and in real-time at the level of a micron scale and automatically quantify these structures provides clinicians with important information about the process of clinical decisions. Among these technological improvements, OCT has a leading role. This technology has been shown to provide reproducible quantification of ocular structures, allowing precise detection of structural damage, monitoring of disease progression, and assessment of the effectiveness of treatment in several retinal pathologies.

Since its first appearance in clinical practice, OCT has evolved substantially with enhancements both in imaging methods and image analysis. These improvements made in the technology have resulted in increased scanning speed, axial and transverse resolution, and more effective use of the OCT technology as a component of multimodal imaging tools. At the same time, the parallel evolution in novel algorithms makes it possible to efficiently analyze more sophisticated data about several ocular diseases from glaucoma disease to retinal and choroidal involvement.

OCT provides high-resolution cross-sectional images of areas of interest using the principle of low-coherence interferometry. The current commercially available generation, SD-OCT, projects a near-infrared broad-bandwidth light to the eye and the frequency information of the back reflected light is used to generate an image. OCT technology is still evolving and it has been shown to be capable of scanning speeds of up to 20.8 million axial scans/second in nonophthalmic applications. Also, the introduction of any OCT improvements like angioOCT techniques will provide us with a better understanding of some pathophysiological behaviors of complicated retinal disease. This represents a new step in understanding the best clinical and surgical approach for several ocular diseases, making us more efficient in terms of prevention and treatment.

This book discusses new developments in OCT technology and its clinical application. It describes some of the most recent advances in OCT technology and techniques for choroidal and retinal diseases. It highlights emerging innovations such as OCT application in the study of macular disease and inherited retinal dystrophy and OCT findings in rare cases such as retinopathy of prematurity. Also, the book provides new insight into the use of OCT in optic nerve diseases, from angioOCT applications for glaucoma and neuro-ophthalmology to a new glance at OCT and glaucoma. Finally, the book discusses miscellaneous uses of OCT.

The applications of these novel OCT systems and techniques will allow closer monitoring of chorioretinal diseases and treatment response, more robust analysis in basic science research, and further insights into surgical management. In addition, these innovations, which optimize visualization of the choroid and retina, offer a promising future for advancing our understanding of the pathophysiology of chorioretinal diseases.

Giuseppe Lo Giudice
San Paolo Ophthalmic Center,
San Antonio Hospital,
University of Padua,
Padova, Italy

Irene Gattazzo
NESMOS Department,
Ophthalmology Unit, St. Andrea Hospital,
University of Rome "La Sapienza",
Rome, Italy

Section 1

Optical Coherence Tomography and Retina

Chapter 1

Role of OCT Angiography OCTA in the Diagnosis of Macular Diseases

Sherin Sadek and Ragai Hatata

Abstract

OCT becomes an indispensable tool in everyday practice. OCTA is the functional extension that provides cross-sectional information on retinal and choroidal circulations without dye injection. It allows visualization of abnormal flow in areas with no flow and abnormal vessels (like CNVM). In ARMD, it can detect active membranes before being leaky in FFA. In diabetic retinopathy, OCTA can diagnose abnormal areas of non-perfusion in the superficial plexus, deeper capillary structures, or neovascularization. OCTA can detect focal dilation and foveal capillaries alterations in macular telangiectasia. It is useful in the diagnosis of inherited retinal diseases such as retinitis pigmentosa. OCTA has many challenges including longer acquisition times and motion artifacts. Longer wavelength SS-OCT may provide a solution for imaging through media opacities and a wider field of view. OCTA does not give full details about the retinal periphery, also, it gives no information about blood-retinal barrier (no dye to leak); an important sign in many retinal diseases.

Keywords: OCTA, macular diseases, retinal circulation, choroidal circulation, CNVM, ARMD

1. Introduction

With the introduction of OCTA, a new era of technological applications in the field of retinal pathologies has been opened. OCTA is a safe, fast imaging tool that allows better delineation of the retinal microvascular and choroidal vascular abnormalities without the risks of dye injection and morbidity hazards. It can show both blood flow and structural changes within the macular area. OCTA also helps to quantify vascular impairment according to the severity of the retinopathy. It is a useful modality for better understanding the real pathology of retinal diseases especially the retinal vascular occlusions, pathological myopia, inherited retinal disorders, and age-related macular degeneration, that opened the way for evaluating the effect of different treatment modalities, and monitoring of disease progression [1]. OCTA, in order to construct a blood flow, compares the differences in the backscattered signal intensity (decorrelation signal) between sequential OCT b-scans taken at a fixed point at a time (representing erythrocyte movement in retinal blood vessels). Incorporation of the split-spectrum amplitude-decorrelation angiography (SSADA) algorithm in flow detection, improves the signal-to-noise ratio. Although OCTA is a rapid three-dimensional scan with many advantages, it has also some limitations including the limited normative database, small field of view, more prone to image artifacts, obscuration by hemorrhage or fluid and the inability to show leakage (FA will remain the gold standard in this) [2]. However, FFA cannot separately visualize the major capillary networks; (superficial retinal, deep retinal, and choriocapillaris) or radial peripapillary network, with the possibility of systemic side effects and allergic reaction to the injected dye. OCTA vascular changes may be affected by the axial length and individuals' systemic vascular risks [3].

NB: A detailed description of OCTA principles was mentioned in the first chapter "OCT from the Past to the Future."

2. OCTA in age-related macular degeneration

Age-related macular degeneration (AMD) is the commonest cause of irreversible visual loss in the elder age group (above 65 years old and more). AMD is classified into two clinically distinct types, that is dry (non-neovascular) AMD and wet (neovascular) AMD. In the former, the clinical hallmark is *drusen* which are yellowish-white deposits within the RPE-Bruch's membrane complex believed to be secondary to metabolic RPE dysfunction as well as impaired conductance of Bruch's membrane. In the clinical course of the disease, dry AMD can either progress to advanced dry AMD with geographic macular atrophy or to wet AMD with the development of choroidal neovascularization which can be sub-RPE (type I), subretinal type II) or intraretinal (type III CNV; also called retinal angiomatous proliferation (RAP).

Different CNV-vessel patterns based on OCTA according to Sulzbacher et al. were assessed. The loose-net (LN) presented as large diameter vessels, well-defined and discernible with a low branching index showing no capillary sprouting. The dense-net (DN) appeared as a hyperreflective vascular net with dense capillary branching. Lesions with a ratio of approximately 50% of areas with large vessel diameter/low branching index and approximately 50% of areas with dense capillary branching were identified as the mixed type. Unidentifiable CNV pattern term was used when no neovascular vessels were detectable (neither in the choriocapillaris CC nor in the outer retina). Darwish classified AMD (according to OCTA lesions) into 2 patterns; pattern I requiring treatment and pattern II not requiring treatment. Pattern I showed all or at least three of the following five features; a well-defined CNV (tortuous lacy-wheel shaped), branching pattern (numerous tiny capillaries), presence of anastomoses and loops, the morphology of the vessel terminals (presence of a peripheral arcade) and perilesional hypo-intense halo. Coscas et al. provided these criteria as a basis for analysis and evaluation of CNV activity and the degree of CNV proliferation, persistence and/or recurrence; conversely, they provide for the stabilization and healing of vessels that become mature or quiescent. While a CNV lesion was considered as pattern II if it showed less than three of the previously reported OCTA features [4–6].

In AMD, OCTA has the advantage of dual appraisal of structural RPE and photoreceptor changes as well as vascular changes of choriocapillaris either choriocapillaris loss in dry AMD or the advent of choroidal neovascular membrane which is the defining feature of wet AMD. The longitudinal correlation between outer retinal and RPE structural changes and choriocapillaris vascular alterations in the clinical context of AMD constitutes the basis for OCTA utility in AMD which serves not only diagnosis but also follow-up and appraisal of response to treatment, for example anti-VEGF (**Figures 1** and 2). However, OCTA choriocapillaris slabs must be assessed cautiously because they are liable to projection and masking artifacts of overlying structures given

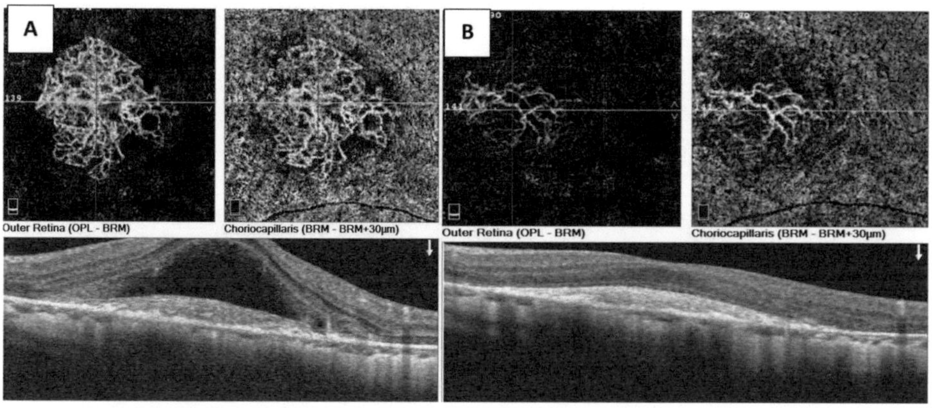

Figure 1.
*A: **Active type 2 CNVM lesion** imaged by Optovue Angiovue OCTA.* **A:** *At the choriocapillaris level, there is a densely packed vascular net formed of loops, and peripheral anastomoses and surrounded by a hypointense halo. The lesion is seen invading the RPE. The B-scan showed accumulated subretinal fluid.* **B:** *After injection, the CNVM shows inactivity. Large mature vessels are seen in a "dead tree" appearance showing no peripheral anastomosis or loops. No fluid accumulation is visible on SD-OCT with macular thinning (atrophy).*

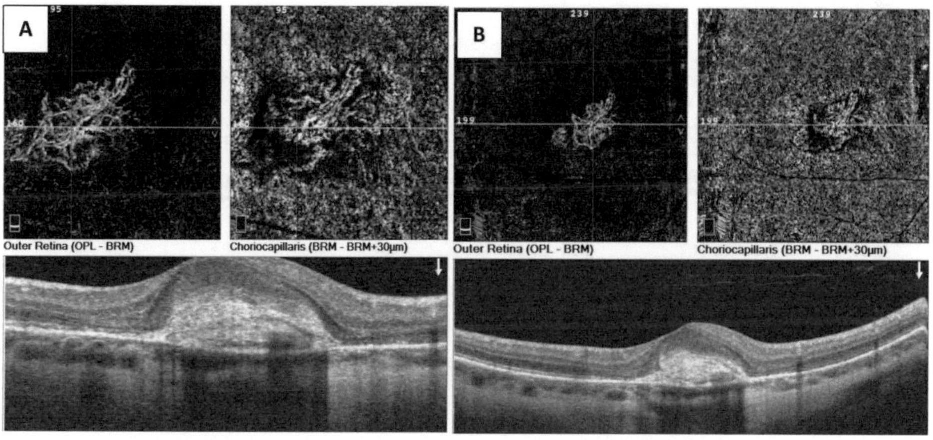

Figure 2.
*A: **Active type 2 CNVM lesion** imaged by Optovue Angiovue OCTA,* **A:** *With a mixed net configuration at choriocapillaris showing minimal activity and increased central thickness in B-scan.* **B:** *After repeated injections, the vascular tree in OCTA gets mature with decreased CMT in SD-OCT scan.*

their deep anatomical location. Therefore, OCTA choriocapillaris slabs must always be correlated with the structural en-face images. OCTA can also show the early subclinical CNV before the signs of activity in the conventional FFA or SD-OCT [7, 8].

3. OCTA in myopic macular-related conditions

Pathological/degenerative myopia is characterized by progressive anteroposterior elongation of the globe with resulting morphological, structural and functional consequences. Ocular pathologies associated with degenerative myopia include myopic traction maculopathy e.g. myopic retinoschisis, posterior staphyloma, parapapillary atrophy, and myopic choroidal neovascular membrane among others. Myopic CNVM has a poor prognosis for central vision preservation and is a major cause of visual morbidity in myopic patients. Since OCTA combines both high-resolution structural B-scans and angiography, it can be useful to demonstrate structural and morphological alterations of myopia like retinoschisis, parapapillary atrophy, dome-shaped macula as well as to detect the development of CNVM (**Figures 3** and **4**). However,

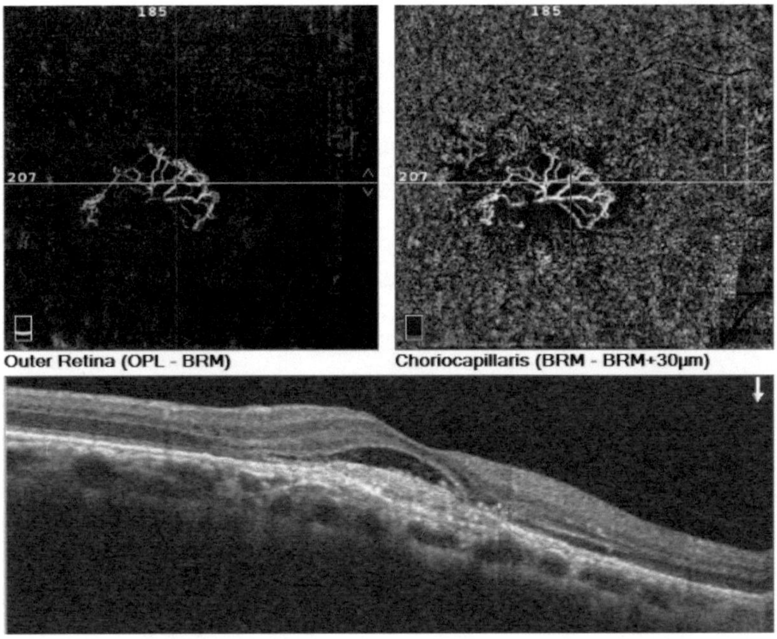

Figure 3.
A myopic CNVM case: *A branching tree with peripheral anastomoses and looping as well as dark halo around the edges conforming activity. The B-scan showed subretinal fluid accumulation denoting activity.*

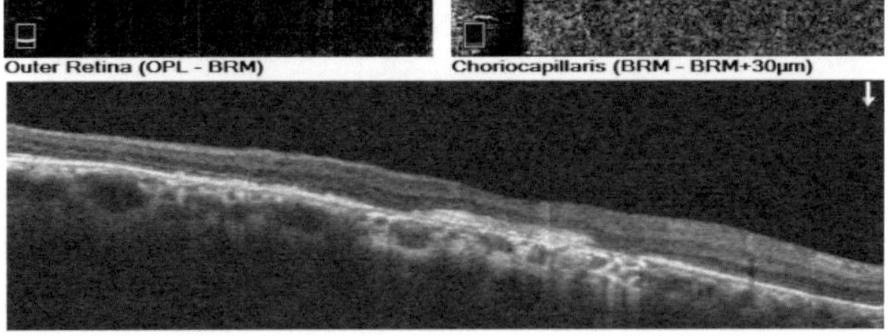

Figure 4.
End-stage myopic CNVM; *a dead tree configuration at the level of choriocapillaris with a lack of branching, anastomoses, and looping.*

the anatomical derangement of the posterior segment in degenerative myopia can pose an obstacle to retrieving high-quality OCTA images with OCTA segmentation artifacts being very common in eyes with degenerative myopia. Therefore, myopic OCTA images have to be examined cautiously and frequently require manual segmentation by an expert to lessen the impact of segmentation artifacts [9, 10].

4. OCTA in macular oedema of different pathologies

Macular oedema is a pathological component of myriad ocular conditions and is a major cause of visual morbidity. Macular oedema can be due to inflammatory cause (as in uveitis), vascular, diabetes mellitus, retinal vein occlusion, CNV, metabolic, or in cases of retinal dystrophies. The high-resolution OCT B-scans allow for accurate description of macular oedema in terms of thickness, morphological pattern (cystoid, spongy or associated neurosensory detachment), and the anatomical involvement of selected retinal layers, the outer plexiform layer (OPL) (**Figure 5**). Such details can be useful not only for disease diagnosis but also for follow-up of treatment response. An advantage of OCTA over the traditional OCT B-scans is the ability to simultaneously correlate macular oedema with the underlying aetiological vascular process, for example ischemia and vascular drop-outs.

In diabetic eyes, OCTA can delineate successfully the enlarged FAZ with underlying non-perfusion that increases according to the severity of diabetic retinopathy, quantitative measurement of vascular density (mainly perfusion density and vessel density), reduced capillary density in the superficial and deep capillary plexuses,

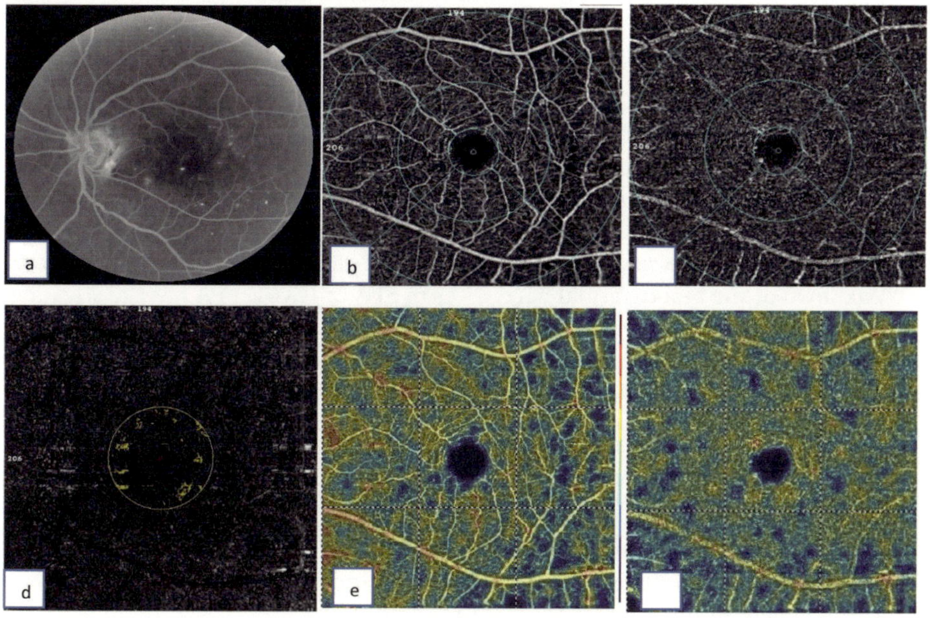

Figure 5.
Optical coherence tomography angiography (OCTA) of mild NPDR with diabetic maculopathy, the SCP (b, e) showed well-defined perifoveal and parafoveal vessels with areas void of flow representing area of capillary drop-outs, more than those seen with the conventional FFA (a). SAME findings in the DCP (c, f) but more advanced regarding the areas of ischemia there is significant decrease in the perfusion as measured by the vessels density and flow index (d) more evident in the DCP.

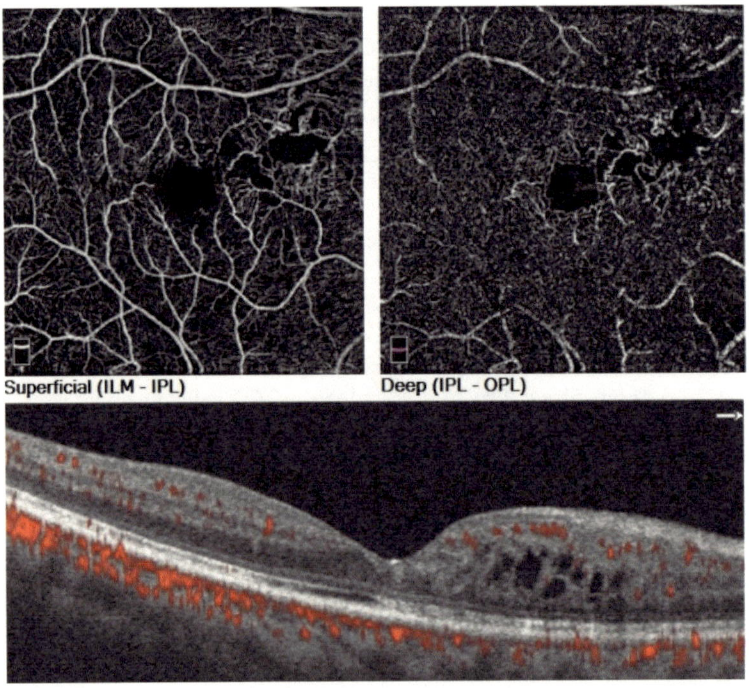

Figure 6.
***Mac Tel type** 2 OCT-angiography shows temporal flow voids areas in the superficial and deep capillary plexuses, spacing between the vessels with increased vascular diameter, and minimal vascular invasion of the FAZ at the deep capillary plexus. The B scan shows multiple hyporeflective cavitations, focal loss of the inner/outer segment with no evidence of external limiting membrane disruption.*

microaneurysms (appear as focally dilated saccular or fusiform capillaries), choriocapillaris flow voids changes and increased vessel tortuosity. Moreover, OCTA may show DR before it is clinically detectable.

However, OCTA has certain limitations in the assessment of vascular retinal diseases associated with macular oedema. It is incapable of testing the structural and functional integrity of vessel walls and hence cannot demonstrate leakage (reflecting the breakdown of the blood-retinal barrier) as in FFA or ICGA. FFA has the advantage of showing abnormal blood vessels, such as retinal neovascularization or intraretinal microvascular abnormalities. In addition, OCTA has so far, a limited imaging field missing most of the peripheral retina which is the main site of pathology in a number of retinal diseases (the developing widefield OCTA technology). Therefore, for DR, fluorescein angiography will remain an essential vital diagnostic modality and OCTA will be the alternative or complementary method of angiography that can be safely (in risky patients especially with impaired kidney functions) and more frequently performed to assess the effectiveness of treatment in DR [11–14].

Macular telangiectasia Type 2 (MacTel2) is a neurodegenerative change affecting the Muller cells in the macular area. SD-OCT abnormalities in MacTel include; cyst formation in the inner retina, disruption of the external limiting membrane, loss of inner/outer segment, parafoveal venular dilation, hyporeflective cavitation of the outer retina, perifoveal capillary leakage, and subretinal neovascularization. In OCTA, Zeimer et al. noted vascular changes in the deep capillary network (enlargement of vessels, larger intervascular spaces, dilated, dendritic appearance

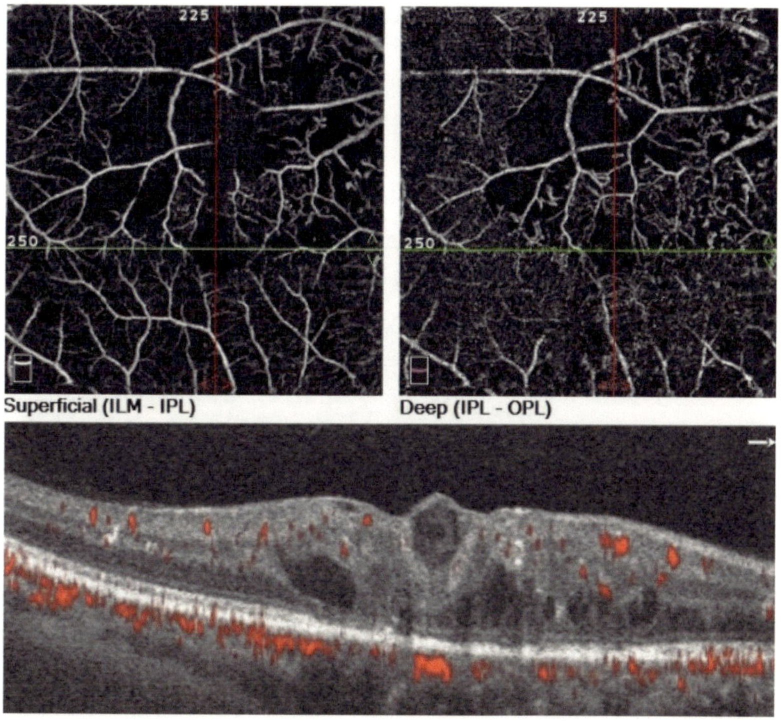

Figure 7.
Advanced mac Tel type 2 *OCT-angiography showed temporal flow voids areas in the superficial and deep capillary plexuses. Telangiectatic vessels are seen among the superficial and deep plexuses with increased vascular diameter as well as rarefied vessels; temporal and superior to the FAZ with right-angled configuration and, vascular invasion of the FAZ at the superficial and deep capillary plexuses. The B scan showed multiple hyporeflective cavitations with focal and diffuse loss of the inner outer segment as well as external limiting membrane disruption.*

of vessels, telangiectasis, reduction and/or loss of capillary density), and the extension of anastomoses toward the superficial capillary network with progression of the disease. RPE-proliferations were often associated with "contraction" of surrounding vessels [14, 15] (**Figures 6** and 7).

5. OCTA in challenging macular disorders

5.1 Vaso-occlusive disorders

Retinal vein occlusions (RVOs) are one of the visually disabling pathologies that lead to impaired capillary perfusion and retinal ischemia. OCTA has the ability to view the retinal vasculature in details as seen in FFA and SD-OCT, which allows accurate evaluation of the microvascular abnormalities including areas of capillary non-perfusion, shunt vessels, vascular dilatation, enlarged the FAZ size, foveal atrophy, intraretinal oedema, and multiple hyporeflective spaces in the inner retinal layers. Bonini Filho et al. reported that OCTA in retinal artery occlusion (RAOs) can accurately delineate retinal capillary plexuses at different levels with the extent of macular ischemia and monitoring vascular flow changes during the disease course [14, 16] (**Figures 8** and **9**).

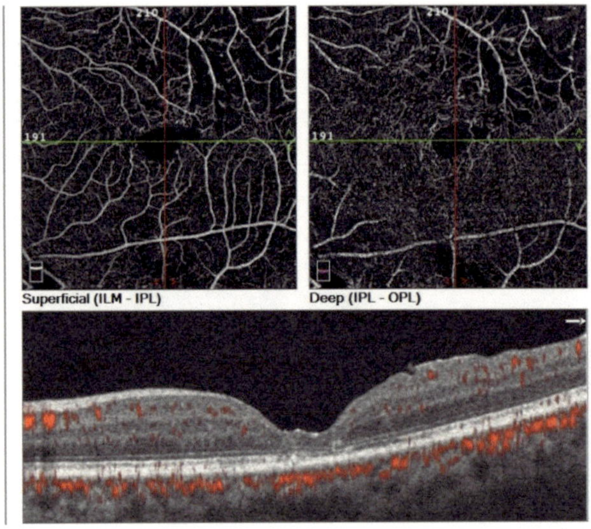

Figure 8.
A case of branch retinal vein occlusion BRVO, OCT-A showed enlarged FAZ with parafoveal flow voids areas in the superficial and deep capillary plexus, more evident in the deep plexus. The b-scan showed interrupted epiretinal membrane with foveal atrophy and multiple hyporeflective spaces in the inner retinal layers. Also, the inner outer photoreceptors segment shows focal disruption up to the ELM.

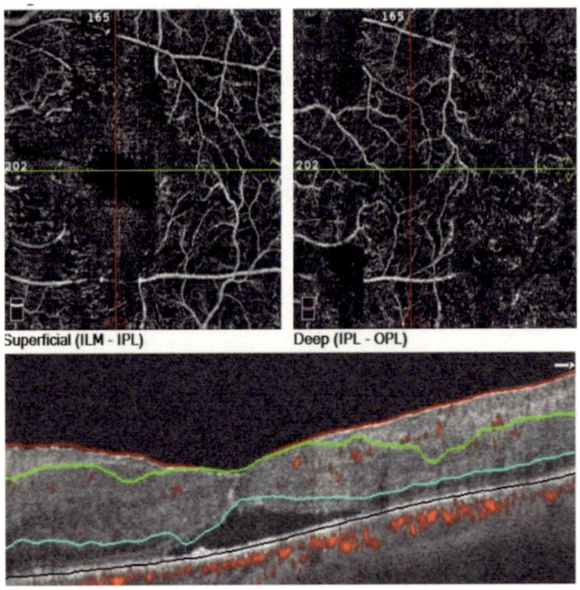

Figure 9.
A case of central retinal vein occlusion CRVO with the OCTA showed asymmetry between the affected and healthy retina. Both superficial and deep network showed rarefied appearance with small telangiectatic vessels at the level of the deep capillary plexus. The RPE and the choriocapillaris showed multiple dark areas representing areas void of flow caused by the shadow casted by the subretinal fluid.

5.2 Inherited retinal dystrophies

Inherited retinal dystrophies are a heterogenous group of diseases that result from mutations in various genes with consequent changes in retinal metabolism that result in photoreceptor loss. The most common retinal dystrophies include vitelliform dystrophy (**Figure 10**), Stargardt's disease (**Figure 11**), and retinitis pigmentosa (**Figure 12**). In Stargardt disease, mutations and subsequent decrease in ABCA4 gene activity results in excessive lipofuscin deposition in RPE. The characteristic dark choroid appearance in FFA of Stargardt results from absorption of the blue excitation light by the lipofuscin pigment in RPE. B-scan OCT in Stargardt disease demonstrates the outer retinal changes of RPE irregularities and shaggy photoreceptor layer with outer retinal loss in the advanced stages. Recently, OCTA showed severe choriocapillaris atrophy coinciding with the areas of RPE and photoreceptor loss that were previously undetectable by FFA due to RPE lipofuscin deposits. Vitelliform dystrophy is due to a mutation in the BEST gene and hence the other name, that is Best disease. In the early stages of the disease, there is progressive deposition of subretinal vitelliform, egg-yolk-colored material, that is vitelliform stage, which then starts to resolve leaving behind variable degrees of photoreceptor loss and may become complicated by CNV. Therefore, OCTA can be very useful to detect the CNV complication of vitelliform dystrophy which is mostly undetectable by either FFA or B-scan OCT due to masking and projection artifacts respectively. Retinitis pigmentosa is an umbrella term for a group of hereditary retinal diseases that share some common clinical and pathological features. Retinitis pigmentosa is historically characterized by the clinical triad of retinal arteriolar attenuation, waxy optic disc pallor, and RPE proliferation and intraretinal migration, which manifest as bone spicule retinal pigmentations. While the main cause of visual impairment in retinitis pigmentosa is photoreceptor loss, other complications may concur and contribute to visual morbidity, for example

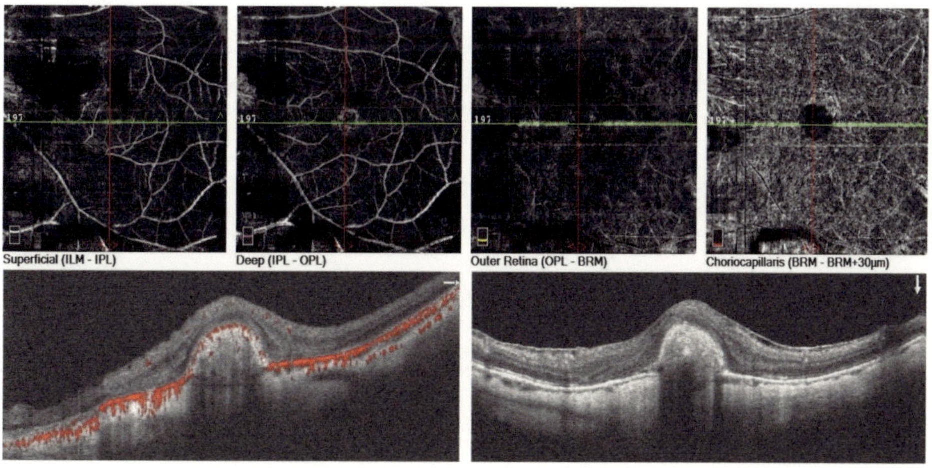

Figure 10.
Adult Vitelliform dystrophy, SD-OCT showed a hyper-reflective material lies between the RPE/Bruch's membrane complex and the photoreceptors layer (ellipsoid zone). In OCTA, there is displacement of blood vessels at the level of the superficial and deep capillary plexus caused by the accumulation of the subretinal material with rarefaction of the choriocapillaris layer.

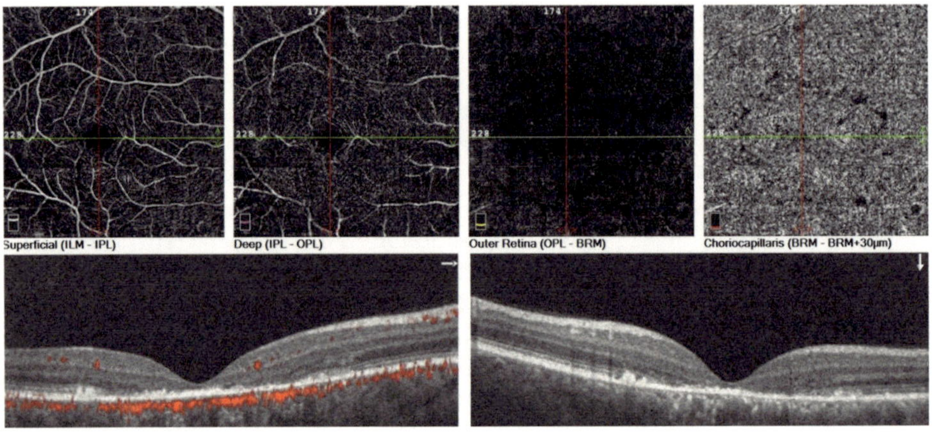

Figure 11.
Stargardt's disease, OCTA showed rarefied superficial and deep capillary plexus with decreased vessel density, decreased flow index, and more exposure of the choroidal blood vessels.

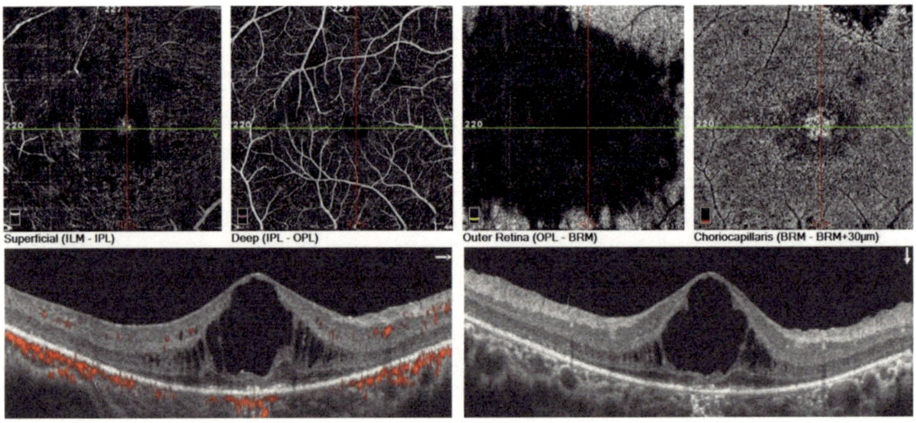

Figure 12.
Retinitis pigmentosa case showed an irregular widened FAZ at the level of the superficial and deep plexus with areas void of flow mainly in the superficial plexus. Diffuse loss at the level of the RPE and the choriocapillaris with exposure of the large choroidal blood vessels findings confirmed by the B-scan showing cystoid oedema and loss of the inner/outer segment as well as the affection of the RPE/choriocapillaris complex.

macular oedema. Consequently, OCTA can prove useful in detecting macular oedema as well as retinal vascular plexus changes in retinitis pigmentosa [17, 18].

The B-scan showed diffuse foveal atrophy with hyperreflective external limiting membrane, loss of the ellipsoid zone, and invariance of retinal tissue through Bruch's membrane.

6. OCTA in inflammatory retinal and uveal diseases

Uveitis is inflammation of the uveal tract, which is the middle vascular coat of the eye. It is classified into anterior, middle, and posterior uveitis according to the anatomical portion involved being the iris and anterior ciliary body, pars plana, and posterior uvea, respectively. While anterior uveitis causes predominantly anterior segment complications, for example cataract, synechia, corneal opacities, and glaucoma; intermediate and posterior uveitis cause posterior segment complications that are the culprits in visual morbidity. Posterior segment complications of uveitis include macular oedema, exudative retinal detachment, CNVM, occlusive retinal vasculitis, and ischemia. Given the major contribution of posterior segment complications in myriad types of uveitis, B-scan OCT and OCTA can be of help in the detection and follow-up of such complications with an accurate characterization of macular oedema, areas of vascular drop-outs, for example ischemia at the different ocular vascular beds, such as the superficial and deep macular vascular plexuses and choriocapillaris. A significant limitation of OCTA in posterior uveitis and retinal vasculitis is the small field of imaging which may not appreciate peripheral retinal involvement which is not only common but also important in proper management like delineating peripheral ischemic retinal zones for subsequent retinal photocoagulation. Therefore, a multimodal imaging approach including wide-field dye-based angiography combined with B-scan OCT and OCTA is a must for proper and comprehensive management of uveitis which mirrors the multidisciplinary approach to uveitis diagnosis [19–21].

7. OCTA in retinal and choroidal tumors

OCTA is an evolving technology that can be useful in the study of posterior segment tumors. The choroidal nevi are mainly seen as heterogenic and hyperreflective lesions. When studying melanocytic tumors, the higher risk of malignancy (choroidal melanoma) is associated with the presence of parilesional hyporeflective plexus or hyperreflective ring (in the choriocapillaris layer) [22] (**Figure 13**).

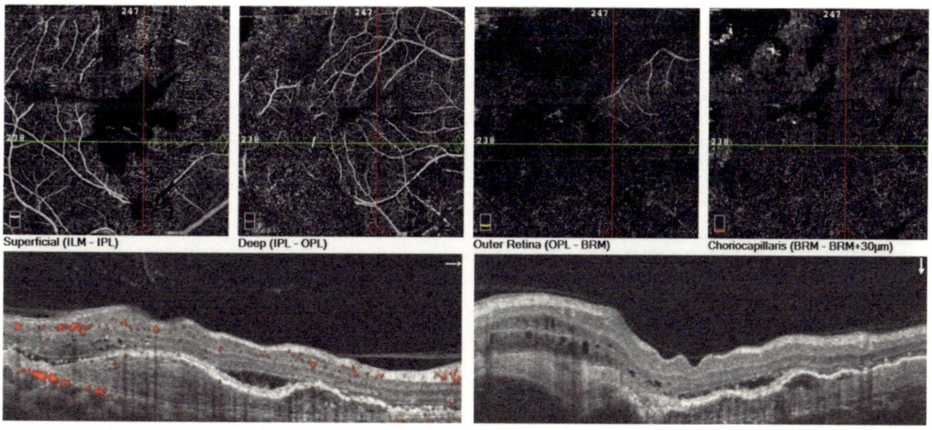

Figure 13.
OCTA of choroidal metastasis, choriocapillaris slab shows significant loss of its' classically mottled appearance, there are areas void of signal indicating tumor invasion of the blood vessel. The b scan showed a classic bumpy appearance with smooth elevation and visible subretinal fluid.

Acknowledgements

Ahmed Ameen Ismail, M.B.B.Ch.
Department of Ophthalmology, Faculty of Medicine, Fayoum University, Al Fayoum, Egypt.

Author details

Sherin Sadek* and Ragai Hatata
Faculty of Medicine-Fayoum University Department of Ophthalmology, Fayoum, Egypt

*Address all correspondence to: sh.sadek@gmail.com; shs00@fayoum.edu.eg

References

[1] Kashani AH, Chen CL, Gahm JK, Zheng F, Richter GM, Rosenfeld PJ, et al. Optical coherence tomography angiography: A comprehensive review of current methods and clinical applications. Progress in Retinal and Eye Research. 2017;**60**:66-100

[2] Carlo T, Romano A, Waheed N, Duker J. A review of optical coherence tomography angiography (OCTA). International Journal of Retina and Vitreous. 2015;**1**:5

[3] Jia Y, Wei E, Wang X, Zhang X, Morrison JC, Parikh M, et al. Optical coherence tomography angiography of optic disc perfusion in glaucoma. Ophthalmology. 2014;**121**:1322-1332

[4] Sulzbacher F, Pollreisz A, Kaider A, Kickinger S, Sacu S, SchmidtErfurth U, et al. Identification and clinical role of choroidal neovascularization characteristics based on optical coherence tomography angiography. Acta Ophthalmologica. 2017;**95**(4):414-420

[5] Darwish A. OCT angiography for the evaluation of wet age related macular degeneration. EC Ophthalmology. 2017;**6**:06-18

[6] Coscas GJ, Lupidi M, Coscas F, Cagini C, Souied EH. Optical coherence tomography angiography versus traditional multimodal imaging in assessing the activity of exudative age-related macular degeneration: A new diagnostic challenge. Retina. 2015;**35**(11):2219-2228

[7] Mitchell P, Liew G, Gopinath B, Wong TY. Age-related macular degeneration. Lancet. 2018;**392**(10153):1147-1159

[8] Ma J, Desai R, Nesper P, Gill M, Fawzi A, Skondra D. Optical coherence tomographic angiography imaging in age-related macular degeneration. Ophthalmology and Eye Diseases. 2017;**9**:117917211668607

[9] Li Y, Zheng F, Foo LL, Wong QY, Ting D, Hoang QV, et al. Advances in OCT imaging in myopia and pathologic myopia. Diagnostics. 2022;**12**:1418

[10] Saw SM, Gazzard G, Shin-Yen EC, Chua WH. Myopia and associated pathological complications. Ophthalmic & Physiological Optics. 2005;**25**(5):381-391

[11] Han R, Gong R, Liu W, Xu G. Optical coherence tomography angiography metrics in different stages of diabetic macular edema. Eye and vision (London, England). 2022;**9**(1):1-9

[12] Khadamy J, Abri Aghdam K, Falavarjani K. An update on optical coherence tomography angiography in diabetic retinopathy. Journal of Ophthalmic & Vision Research. 2018;**13**(4):487

[13] Chua J, Sim R, Tan B, Wong D, Yao X, Liu X, et al. Optical coherence tomography angiography in diabetes and diabetic retinopathy. Journal of Clinical Medicine. 2020;**9**(6):1723

[14] Chalam K, Sambhav K. Optical coherence tomography angiography in retinal diseases. Journal of Ophthalmic & Vision Research. 2016;**11**(1):84-92. DOI: 10.4103/2008-322X.180709

[15] Zeimer M, Gutfleisch M, Heimes B, Spital G, Lommatzsch A, Pauleikhoff D. Association between changes in macular vasculature in optical coherence tomography- and fluorescein – Angiography and distribution of macular

pigment in type 2 idiopathic macular telangiectasia. Retina. 2015;**35**:2307-2316

[16] Bonini Filho MA, Adhi M, de Carlo TE, Ferrara D, Baumal CR, Witkin AJ, et al. Optical coherence tomography angiography in retinal artery occlusion. Retina. 2015;**35**:2339-2346

[17] Liu G, Liu X, Li H, Du Q, Wang F. Optical coherence tomographic analysis of retina in retinitis Pigmentosa patients. Ophthalmic Research. 2016;**56**(3):111-122

[18] Parodi MB, Arrigo A, Bandello F. Optical coherence tomography angiography quantitative assessment of macular neovascularization in best vitelliform macular dystrophy. Investigative Ophthalmology & Visual Science. 2020;**61**(6):61-61

[19] Agarwal A, Invernizzi A. The Role of Optical Coherence Tomography and Optical Coherence Tomography Angiography in the Differential Diagnosis of Posterior Uveitis. Ocular Immunology and Inflammation. 3 Apr 2022;**30**(3):682-689

[20] Invernizzi A, Cozzi M, Staurenghi G. Optical coherence tomography and optical coherence tomography angiography in uveitis: A review. Clinical & Experimental Ophthalmology. 2019;**47**(3):357-371

[21] Marchese A, Agarwal A, Moretti AG, Handa S, Modorati G, Querques G, et al. Advances in imaging of uveitis. Therapeutic Advances in Ophthalmology. 2020;**12**:251584142091778

[22] Toledo J, Asencio M, García J, Morales L, Tomkinson C, Cajigal C. OCT angiography: Imaging of choroidal and retinal tumors. Ophthalmology Retina. 2018;**2**(6):613-622

Chapter 2

OCT from the Past to the Future

Sherin Sadek and Ragai Hatata

Abstract

OCT is a high-resolution, non-invasive imaging technique that relies on time-of-flight information. Different patterns such as time domain and spectral domain were implemented until the introduction of the longer wavelength new generation, swept-source OCT. Anterior segment OCT has different implications as AC angle assessment, tear meniscus measurement, corneal pathologies, etc. In posterior segment, macular lesions are easier to image (vitreoretinal interface, intraretinal changes, subretinal and choroidal pathologies). OCT-ON is an important tool in investigating glaucoma and optic neuropathies. Recent advances made OCT indispensable tool in everyday practice. Functional extension providing information on retinal and choroidal circulations without the need for dye injection is the OCT angiography. ONH-OCTA and AS-OCTA imaging vasculature are useful for various clinical applications, ranging from diagnosis to treatment with many challenges. Major advances occurred in the intraoperative OCT, from portable probe to the microscope-integrated system and handheld type. Developing technologies are coming as doppler OCT, in-vivo retinal images and polarization-sensitive OCT.

Keywords: OCT, time-domain, spectral domain, swept source, intraoperative OCT

1. Introduction

Optical coherence tomography (OCT) is a high-resolution, cross-sectional imaging technique. It is fast, safe and non-invasive modality. Over the past 25 years, OCT has advanced to become the most commonly used investigative tool in ophthalmology. The 3D imaging allows qualitative and quantitative structural analysis of different locations in the retina and optic nerve head. It helps not only to improve the diagnosis but also to understand the pathogenesis of various diseases and to evaluate the effect of the implemented therapies.

2. Evolution of OCT technology

Originally, OCT technology was used to localize faults in fiber optic networks in the telecommunications industry [1]. A back light was reflected from a disruption in a fibreoptic cable, and the time-of-flight information was extracted by low-coherence interferometry to enable distance mapping [2]. OCT was introduced in ophthalmology in 1991 as an application of low-coherence interferometry used in axial length measurement [3]. Other developments that added much to the industry of OCT were semi-conductor, super-luminescent diode SLD (low cost and low maintenance light source), optical heterodyne detection (improving safe detection and interpretation of faint signals) and high-speed line camera technology (incorporating fast repetitive A-scans to give the 2D images "B-scan"). Then, James Fujimoto and his coworkers were the first to represent brightness by employment of the color codes [2].

The first commercially available OCT device was by Zeiss in 1996 after the scanning patterns with reproducible measurements were implemented. In 2000, the second OCT generation was fairly acceptable in ophthalmology practice due to slow speed (100 axial scans/second) and low resolution [2]. Then, the speed was increased in 2002 to 400 axial scans in the third-generation devices for scanning of the anterior segment, retinal layers and optic nerve, and these A-scans became incorporated into a commercial system with an axial resolution of ~10 μm^2 [4]. In 2006, the faster Fourier domain approach using 27,000 A-scans/second was introduced (RTVue, OptoVue, USA).

The adaptive optics AO to correct the ocular monochromatic aberrations was first reported in OCT by Miller et al. in 2003 improving the transverse resolution [5]. However, this AO had a narrow depth of focus that prevented simultaneous visualization of layers at different depths and restricted field of view.

The polarization sensitive was used in OCT in 2001 to measure birefringence of the RNFL of the monkeys [6], and then later on, it was used for birefringence measurement of the retina and anterior segment.

3. OCT: basic principles and preclinical application

OCT is a type of "optical ultrasound" as it relies on time-of-flight information, similar to the ultrasound. It is like an in-vivo optical biopsy analyzing the signals from different locations at different depths [7]. The OCT resolution fills the gap between the ultrasound and conofocal microscopy resolutions.

Light interference is the core principle in OCT imaging based on the optical fiber-based Michelson setup. When the light emits from a low-coherence source, it will split by a coupler into two parts traveling to both arms, namely sample and reference arms. To control different beam parameters (as shape, depth of focus and intensity distribution), the light emitted from the fiber end of either arm is shaped by various optical components (mirrors, lenses, etc.). The backscattered light from both arms will pass through the coupler to be recorded by the detector (**Figure 1**). The difference in the light backscattered from the sample arm will exit when it encounters an interface

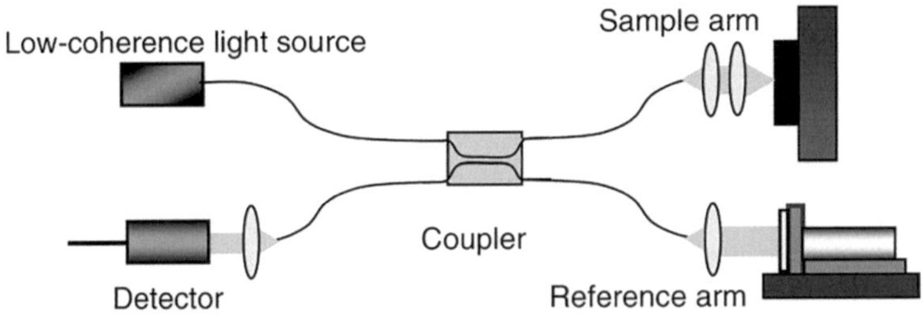

Figure 1.
Optical fiber-based Michelson setup demonstrating the basic concept of light interference in OCT imaging (figure taken from Popescu et al. [8]).

between structures of different refractive indices. The corresponding interference pattern is formed between the light propagating in the reference arm traveled a certain optical distance and the light that traveled the same optical distance along the sample arm (including the portion of the distance traveled inside the sample). The depth information of light backscattered from the locations of various structures within the sample can be measured in this way. The detector records the OCT signal during a complete travel of the reference mirror "Depth or A-scan" which is recorded at each beam position. While the B-scan is formed by a consecutive set of A-scans [8].

The 3D imaging allows not only analysis from different locations but also incorporation of A-scans to form the OCT fundus (en face) image [4]. This is called full-field OCT (FF-OCT) with an axial resolution of ~1 μm^2, similar to that of the conventional microscopy [8]. Also, the built-in tracking system allows better sensitivity and higher reproducibility.

In OCT imaging, the axial and transverse resolutions are independent. The axial resolution (depth resolution and coherence gate) is the coherence length of the source which is inversely proportional to its bandwidth. Therefore, broadband optical sources are required to achieve high axial resolution. While the transverse resolution is determined by the minimum spot size of the focused probing beam (inversely proportional to the numerical aperture NA of the focusing lens). This transverse resolution affects the depth of field (a low NA with a greater beam diameter will offer a large depth of field, as in most OCT imaging). The transverse resolutions used by the commercially available OCT systems are between 20 and 25 μm^2 [8]. The lateral resolution is considered to be equal to the illumination spot size on the retina (14 μm for Spectralis OCT) [9].

4. First clinical applications and the early diagnostic efficacy

The time-domain (TD)-OCT imaging was firstly developed in 1990s. It included 3.4 mm scan around the optic nerve head and six radial scans (6 mm) at the macula for assessment of glaucoma, optic neuropathies and retinal diseases [4]. Then, the introduction of the 3D approaches allowed the imaging of ganglion cell complex GCC, RNFL thickness map, comparison to a normal population and comparison of different scans over time for detection of any subtle structural changes reflecting the disease progression. Also, the progression in OCT development allowed better thickness measurements, analysis of the vitreoretinal interface and detection of biomarkers as predictors of the surgical outcome and visual prognosis.

Anterior segment AS-OCT is a non-contact imaging device that provides the detailed structure of the anterior part of the eye including the cornea and anterior chamber angle. It is beneficial in presurgical and postsurgical assessment of corneal and lenticular refractive surgeries. Unlike ultrasound biomicroscopy UBM, it does not allow visualization of the ciliary body.

5. Time domain vs. Fourier domain

5.1 Advantages and disadvantage

TD-OCT uses low coherence interferometry with the light being split to be sent to both a scanning reference mirror and the sample. The interference occurs when the reflected beams recombine. The intensity information can be extracted from the

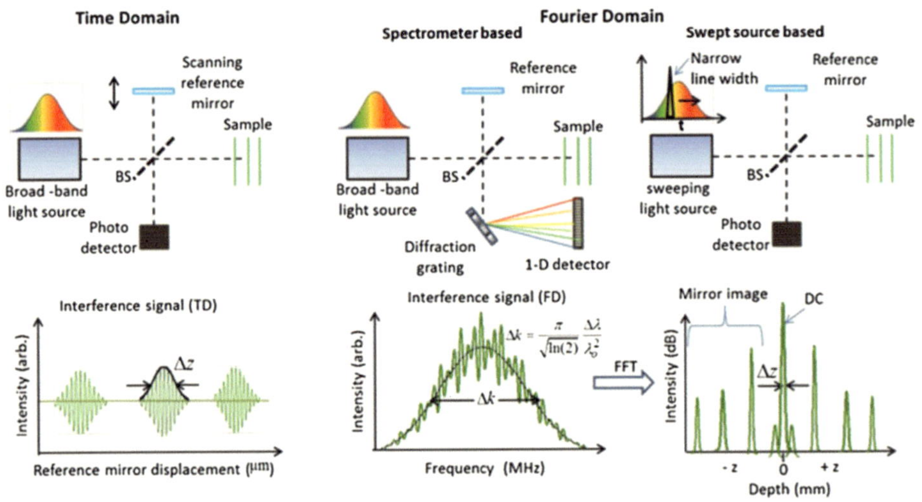

Figure 2.
Principles of different approaches of OCT, time domain versus Fourier domain (figure is taken from Wolfgang et al. [10]).

interference profile. Different depths in the tissue sample can be scanned by changing the location of the reference mirror [4]. The TD-OCT approach encodes the location reflections and relates them to the position of the moving reference mirror, and the time-encoded signals are recorded sequentially. It is limited by the slow-scan acquisition time and 2D imaging with an axial resolution of ~10 μm^2 [2] (**Figure 2**).

The A-scans in the other approach are obtained using a Fourier transform of the detected frequencies. It uses a single axial scan by evaluating spectrum of interference between stationary reference mirror and reflected light. The light echoes come at the same time from all axial depths with simultaneous capture of all the spectral components, hence the advantages of improving 3D scan resolution with an axial resolution of ~2-5 μm^2 and reducing the acquisition time up to 27,000–100,000 A-scans/second9. The Fourier domain includes both the spectral domain (SD) and the swept-source (SS)-OCT. In the SD-OCT approach, a broad-bandwidth light source, charge-coupled device (CCD) camera and a spectrometer are used to acquire frequency information, while the SS-OCT is sweeping a narrow band through broad range with a photodetector [2] (**Figure 3**). The limits of pixels of CCD camera and the dispersed interference pattern immediately before detection are drawbacks of SD over SS-OCT, while the SS-OCT has the advantages of point detection, less movement artifacts, better signal-to-noise ratio with better visualization of different retinal and choroidal pathologies [4, 8] (**Figure 3**).

5.2 The swept-source technology

It is a unique combination of high speed, deep tissue penetration and high-resolution OCT technology. It allows simultaneous visualization of the vitreous, retina and choroid. Visualization of choroidal structure may play a role in understating the pathogenesis of retinal diseases. Presenting the optic nerve and macula on the same scan is possible with its wide scans. Longer wavelengths are beneficial in eyes with hazy fundus view due to media opacity as in cataractous eyes [12].

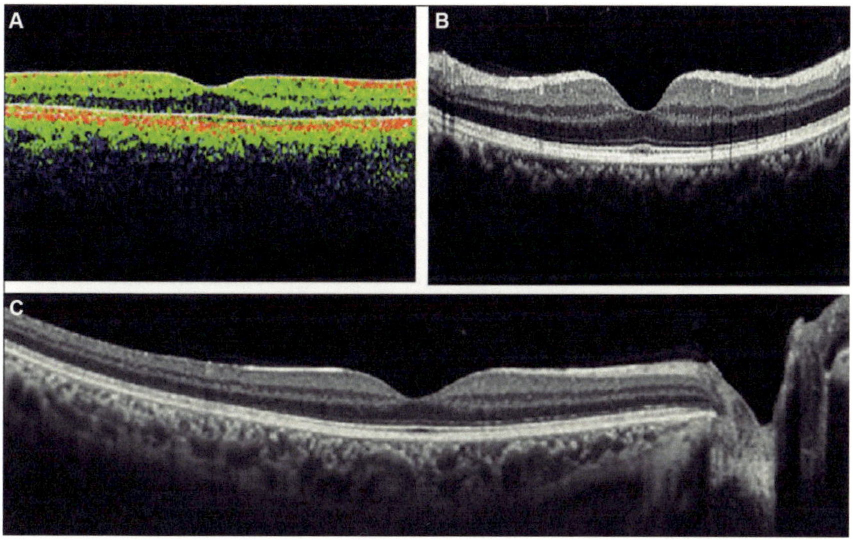

Figure 3.
Normal OCT-macula as captured by A: Time-domain OCT, B: Spectral domain OCT and C: Swept source OCT [11].

The advantage in SS-OCT performance is due to the laser source performance (a wavelength-swept laser). The advances in development of several types of wavelength-swept lasers improve the speed and depth of imaging and eliminating the mechanical movement (active mode-locking (AML) laser) [13].

6. Developing technologies

Longer wavelengths OCT systems for better visualization of the choroid and retina are emerging. Major advances occur in the intraoperative iOCT; from a handheld portable probe used in infants and bed-ridden patients (it was used firstly in patient undergoing vitrectomy for better visualization of the macular disease [4]) to the microscope-integrated system (firstly demonstrated in the anterior segment surgeries) guiding the image during ophthalmic surgeries.

OCT-slit lamp incorporation also is advancing for close monitoring of chorioretinal diseases. The visible-light (Vis) OCT technology develops to capture retinal fine details. FF-OCT provides 2D enface high resolution images at different depth. The wide-field (WF) and ultrawide-field (UWF) increases the field of imaging to 40–55 degrees in WF up to 200 degrees in UWF allowing visualization of the periphery.

The AO-OCT improves the quality of images by using wavefront component and advanced software to compensate the ocular aberrations. At-home OCT is a self-imaging technique for better monitoring of the disease when compared to the in-office imaging.

Polarization-sensitive OCT analyses the tissue polarization and depolarization quantitively of the retinal pigment epithelial layers. Doppler OCT and, In-vivo retinal images developing technologies are coming [14].

7. OCTA introduction and the future of FFA

Over the past years, OCT was used to assess the structural anatomy (3D) of the posterior segment, while fluorescein angiography (FA) was used to assess the retinal vasculature (2D). Then, optical coherence tomography angiography (OCTA) develops since 2014 to represent the functional extension of structural OCT that allows non-invasive visualization and qualification of the retinal and choroidal microcirculations, without the need for dye injections. Also, OCTA shows developmental progression in earlier diagnosis of glaucoma and neuro-ophthalmology diseases. OCTA decreases the use of the invasive FA especially after the diagnosis [15].

The main principle of OCTA is the detection of signal change over time emitted from intravascular blood cells motions. The scan consists of multiple individual A-scans using the laser light reflected from the surface of moving red blood cells, which integrated into a B-scan providing cross-sectional information (**Figure 4**). There are two methods used for motion detection: amplitude decorrelation (differences in amplitude between two different B-scan) or phase variance (the variation of phase of the emitted light wave when it intercepts moving objects). The same tissue area is repeatedly imaged, analyzing the differences between scans to differentiate between areas of high flow and that of slow/no flow [16]. The signals are amplified with different motion correction technologies aiming to improve the image quality.

OCTA machines are characterized by autosegmentation which referred to splitted slabs from a known anatomical layer of the retinal vasculature. In Optovue OCTA software, the four slabs represent the following: superficial capillary plexus SCP, deep capillary plexus DCP, outer retina and choriocapillaris as shown in **Figure 5**. While the SCP is seen on FA, the DCP is poorly seen on FA and hence the advantage of OCTA in diagnosis of certain pathological conditions as retinal angiomatous proliferation, paracentral acute middle maculopathy and parafoveal telangectasia. The outer retinal slab is useful in identification of type 2 (subretinal) neovascular membranes, while the choriocapillaris slab helps to detect early type 1 (sub-RPE) choroidal neovascular membrane (CNV) [15].

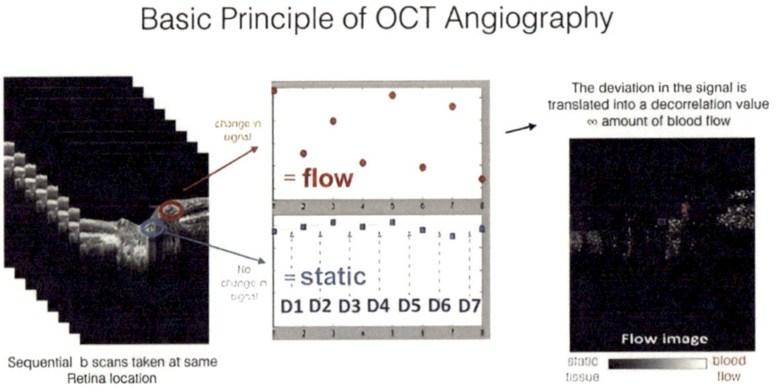

Figure 4.
Basic principle of optical coherence tomography angiography; when the B-scans are sequentially taken from the same retinal location, any changes in signal amplitude or phase will represent the blood flow, and mathematical assessment of signal changes will represent the amount of the blood flow [15].

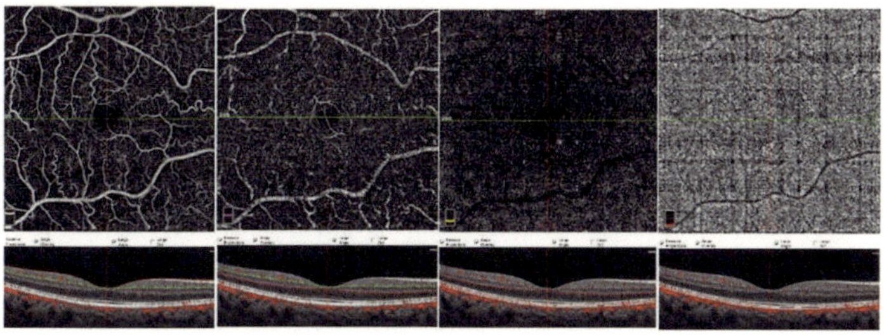

Figure 5.
Optovue OCTA four slabs; a: Inner retinal slab extends from 3 μm below the internal limiting membrane (ILM) to 15 μm below the inner plexiform layer (IPL) representing the superficial retinal vascular plexus. B: Middle retinal slab representing the deep capillary plexus; extends from 15 μm below the IPL to 70 μm below the IPL. C: Outer retinal slab showing no vessels in normal individuals, extends from 70 μm below the IPL to 30 μm below the retinal pigment epithelium (RPE). D: The last slab represents the choriocapillaris extending from 30 μm below the RPE to 60 μm below the RPE.

OCTA device	Used technology	Advantages
1. ZEISS Angioplex™ OCT angiographic imaging on the CIRRUS™ HD-OCT platform	FastTrac™ software	Scanning rate up to 68,000 A-scans per second.
2. Optovue AngioVue® (Optovue, Inc., Freemont, CA)	Split-spectrum amplitude-decorrelation angiography algorithm (SSADA)	Minimizes motion Noise, allows quantitative Analysis of flow area and flow density maps.
3. Topcon®	OCTA RatioAnalysis paired with SD-OCT	Reduces motion artifacts, Preserves axial resolution Improves detection sensitivity of low blood flow
4. Heidelberg engineering®	Active eye-tracking system (TruTrack™)	Simultaneously acquisition of fundus and OCT images for better signal-to-noise ratio.

Table 1.
Main commercially available devices of OCT-A [16].

Variable interscan time analysis (VISTA) allows visualization of different ranges of blood flow speeds using a color-encoded images in which high flow is represented in red color and blue represents areas of relatively low flow.

OCTA provides images of blood cell movements (perfusion) and not anatomical structure of the vessels. Areas of ischemia are represented as dark zones. There are different chorioretinal pathologies that can be diagnosed using OCTA; abnormal flow in areas with no flow (like presence of CNV in the outer retina), abnormal areas of non-perfusion in the SCP (normally there is a foveal avascular zone in the center) with an extension of the non-perfused area as in diabetic retinopathy.

There are many challenges in OCTA that are tried to be corrected by various technologies as shown in **Table 1** (as longer data acquisition times needed for repeated B-scans, corrected by SSADA, motion artifacts corrected by dual track technology). We should note that OCTA does not give us full details about retinal periphery, and also, it gives no information about blood retinal barrier (no dye to leak), an important sign in many retinal diseases. Some limitations and artifacts are also important to consider in the OCT-A images interpretation.

8. Conclusion

This introduction chapter gives a brief review about the history of development of OCT. OCT is a non-invasive revolutionary imaging modality with vast growing technology. Starting from the past, the progression in wavelengths, sensitivity, reproducibility and decrease scan acquisition time are evolving. Recent advances in technology make OCT indispensable tool in everyday practice and accepted as the standard of care. OCTA is giving new information that FA and ICGA cannot provide. iOCT and handheld models are considered the next big step in OCT development.

Conflict of interest

The authors declare no conflict of interest.

Author details

Sherin Sadek* and Ragai Hatata
Faculty of Medicine, Ophthalmology Department, Fayoum University, Fayoum, Egypt

*Address all correspondence to: sh.sadek@gmail.com; shs00@fayoum.edu.eg

References

[1] Takada K, Yokohama I, Chida K, Noda J. New measurement system for fault location in optical waveguide devices based on an interferometric technique. Applied Optics. 1987;**26**: 1603-1606

[2] Kothari AR. Optical Coherence Tomography-Evolution and Clinical Applications. Jaipur, Rajasthan: eOphtha; 2021. Available from: https://www.eophtha.com/posts/optical-coherence-tomography-evolution-and-clinical-applications

[3] Fercher AF, Mengedoht K, Werner W. Eye-length measurement by interferometry with partially coherent light. Optics Letters. 1988;**13**:186-188. DOI: 10.1364/ol.13.000186

[4] Gabriele ML, Wollstein G, Ishikawa H, Kagemann L, Juan X, Folio LS, et al. Optical coherence tomography: History, current status, and laboratory work. Investigative Ophthalmology & Visual Science. 2011;**52**(5):2425-2436. DOI: 10.1167/iovs.10-6312

[5] Miller DT, Kocaoglu OP, Wang Q, Lee S. Adaptive optics and the eye (super resolution OCT). Eye (Lond). Mar 2011;**25**(3):321-330. DOI: 10.1038/eye.2011.1. PMID: 21390066; PMCID: PMC3113555

[6] Ducros MG, Marsack JD, Rylander HG 3rd, Thomsen SL, Milner TE. Primate retina imaging with polarization-sensitive optical coherence tomography. Journal of the Optical Society of America. A, Optics, Image Science, and Vision. 2001;**18**:2945-2956

[7] Choma M, Sarunic M, Yang C, Izatt J. Sensitivity advantage of swept source and Fourier domain optical coherence tomography. Optics Express. 2003;**11**:2183-2189. DOI: 10.1364/OE.11.002183

[8] Popescu D, Choo-Smith L, Flueraru C, Mao Y, Chang S, Disano J, et al. Optical coherence tomography: Fundamental principles, instrumental designs and biomedical applications. Biophysical Reviews. 2011;**3**(3):155. DOI: 10.1007/s12551-011-0054-7

[9] Spaide RF, Otto T, Caujolle S, Kübler J, Aumann S, Fischer J, et al. Lateral resolution of a commercial optical coherence tomography instrument. Translational Vision Science & Technology. 2022;**11**(1):28. DOI: 10.1167/tvst.11.1.28

[10] Drexler W, Liu M, Kumar A, Kamali T. Optical coherence tomography today: Speed, contrast, and multimodality. Journal of Biomedical Optics. 2014;**19**(7):71412. DOI: 10.1117/1.JBO.19.7.071412

[11] Bhende M, Shetty S, Parthasarathy M, Ramya S. Optical coherence tomography: A guide to interpretation of common macular diseases. Indian Journal of Ophthalmology. Jan 2018;**66**(1):20-35

[12] Michalewska Z, Michalewski J, Nawrocki J. Swept-source OCT wide-field simultaneous choroid, retina, and vitreous visualization. Retina Today. 2013:50-56

[13] Park KS, Park E, Lee H, et al. Phase stable swept-source optical coherence tomography with active mode-locking laser for contrast enhancements of retinal angiography. Scientific Reports. 2021;**11**:16636. DOI: 10.1038/s41598-021-95982-9

[14] Ong J, Zarnegar A, Corradetti G, Singh S, Chhablani J. Advances in optical coherence tomography imaging technology and techniques for choroidal and retinal disorders. Journal of Clinical Medicine. 2022;**11**:5139. DOI: 10.3390/jcm11175139

[15] Optical Coherence Tomography Angiography: Understanding the Basics. Website: https://entokey.com/optical-coherence-tomography-angiography-understanding-the-basics/

[16] O'Keefe G, Breda J, Tripathy K, Sousa D, Pinto L, Palestine A, et al. Optical Coherence Tomography Angiography. A Service of the American Academy of Ophthalmology, EyeWiki; 2022

Chapter 3

New OCT and OCTA Insights in Inherited Retinal Dystrophies

Alessandro Arrigo, Lorenzo Bianco, Alessio Antropoli, Andrea Saladino, Alessandro Berni, Maurizio Battaglia Parodi and Francesco Bandello

Abstract

Optical coherence tomography (OCT) and OCT angiography (OCTA) radically changed the diagnostics of inherited retinal dystrophies (IRD), providing new information regarding the microstructural changes occurring in each disease. The introduction of quantitative metrics provided even more steps forward in the understanding of IRD pathogenesis and course, allowing to propose new ways to categorize different subgroups of patients, characterized by remarkably different characteristics and prognosis. All these informations provided insights regarding how heterogeneous the clinical spectrum of IRD is. In the present study, we provide an updated description of OCT and OCTA findings in the main IRD, including retinitis pigmentosa, Stargardt disease, and Best vitelliform macular dystrophy. Moreover, we discuss imaging findings in pigmented paravenous retinochoroidal atrophy, a rare condition that is undergoing even growing scientific and clinical interest. In addition, we provided a brief updated scenario on imaging findings in pattern dystrophies. We discuss in detail the current state-of-the-art and the new insights provided by quantitative OCT and OCTA approaches, offering a complete description that might be helpful both for expert and nonexpert researchers interested in IRD.

Keywords: OCT, OCTA, IRD, STGD, RP, BVMD, PPCRA, pattern dystrophy

1. Introduction

Inherited retinal dystrophies (IRD) represent a group of extremely heterogeneous retinal disorders. In recent years, several steps forward in the understanding of IRD pathogeneses and clinical courses have been provided by the use of quantitative multimodal retinal imaging, namely a set of noninvasive diagnostic techniques allowing to reach a very high, histology-like level of details. The main multimodal retinal imaging technologies are based on fundus autofluorescence (FAF), optical coherence tomography (OCT), and OCT angiography (OCTA), although many other ancillary techniques are even more employed both in research and clinical contexts [1]. The combined use of these imaging modalities allows to obtain highly detailed information regarding the morphological and biochemical properties of retinal diseases.

The even larger use of multimodal retinal imaging provided undoubted advantages in retinal diagnostics, and IRD highly benefitted from this, watching the increasing interest of research groups and companies in developing new treatment strategies [2]. From this point of view, the next years will provide meaningful changes regarding the management of IRD, providing new potential treatments and changing the clinical course of these genetically determined retinal diseases. These are the reason why ophthalmologists and retinal specialists should be more focused on reaching a good level of knowledge regarding IRD imaging findings, especially looking at OCT and OCTA ones. The main goal of this chapter is to provide an updated and complete scenario regarding OCT and OCTA characteristics of the most common IRD, namely retinitis pigmentosa (RP), Stargardt disease (STGD), and Best vitelliform macular dystrophy (BVMD). In addition, we dedicated a section to pigmented paravenous retinochoroidal atrophy (PPCRA), a rare retinal disorder characterized by still unknown pathogenesis, which is currently an object of very high research interest. A brief description regarding the current literature findings in pattern dystrophies is also provided.

2. Retinitis pigmentosa

RP is the most common IRD form, characterized by very high genotypical and phenotypical heterogeneity [3]. RP is a progressive, centripetal disease characterized by primary damage of rod photoreceptors followed by cone photoreceptors involvement in later stages [3]. The clinical presentation is mainly characterized by night blindness and peripheral visual field alterations; central vision impairment occurs in more advanced stages of the disease. The classic fundoscopic triad is made by optic disc pallor, attenuated retinal vessels, and "bone-spicule" peripheral retinal pigment deposits. A complete noninvasive multimodal retinal imaging RP case is shown in **Figure 1**.

FAF examination is characterized by peripheral diffuse hypoautofluorescence. The central retina is surrounded by the typical Robson-Holder hyperautofluorescence ring, interpreted as RPE reactive phenomenon correlating with the integrity of the outer retinal bands and the progression of the disease [4, 5]. The central retina may be characterized by different amount of FAF alterations, depending on the status of the outer retina and the occurrence of macular edema. FAF deterioration was found strictly related with the electrophysiology evidence of retinal functional decline [4].

OCT provided undoubtedly advantages in detecting the changes occurring at the level both of inner and outer retinal layers. It offers the most detailed representation of the status of outer retinal bands, correlating with visual acuity, retinal sensitivity, and RP progression [6]. In particular, the status of an external limiting membrane (ELM), ellipsoid zone (EZ), outer nuclear layer (ONL), and outer hyperreflective bands ruled the central vision and peripheral visual field [7, 8]. Electrophysiology investigations also highlighted a relationship between the integrity and thickness of inner retinal layers and the functionality of the central retina [9]. Many times, myopia-related alterations coexist with typical signs of retinal degeneration related to RP [10]. In advanced stages, outer retinal tubulations (ORT) can be identified on structural OCT [10]. ORT is defined as round outer retinal structures with hyperreflective borders surrounding a mixed reflectivity core, usually located at the borders of, or centrally within, regions of outer retinal atrophy [11]. ORT formation is made by the gradual remodeling and invagination of the ELM-photoreceptors complex and is commonly interpreted as a degenerative sign. Although RP is mainly considered an outer retinal disorder, even growing evidence are suggesting a major involvement

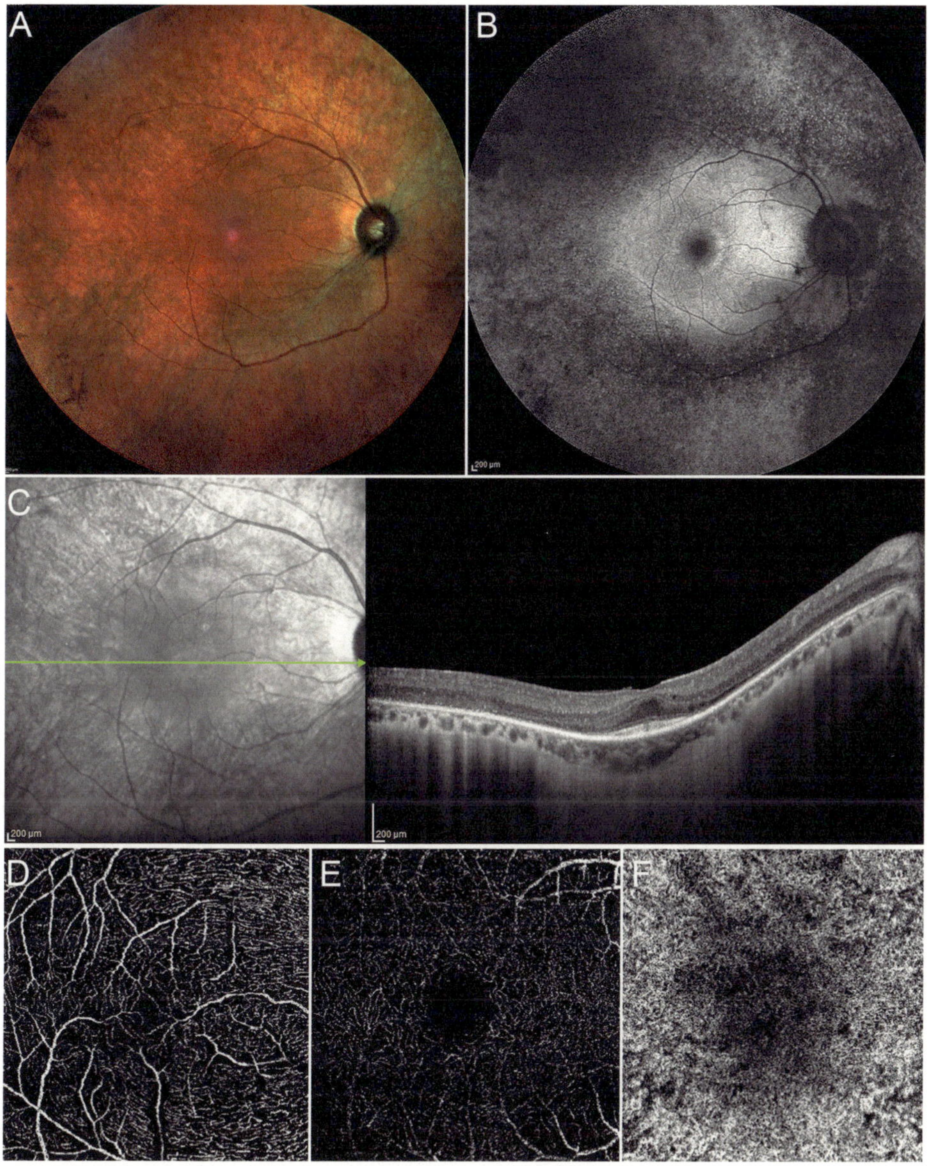

Figure 1.
Multimodal retinal imaging in RP. Confocal multicolor image (A) shows changes in the peripheral pigment with some bone spicule, attenuated retinal vasculature, and central pigment rarefaction. FAF image (B) shows extensive peripheral hypoautofluorescent signal, the perifoveal hyperautofluorescent Robson-Holder ring, and the preserved central physiological hypoautofluorescence. Structural OCT (C) shows the disappearance of the peripheral outer retinal bands, with preservation limited to the foveal region. Moreover, OCT shows myopic signs, such as the increased curvature of the eye and thin choroid. OCTA shows preserved SCP (D), markedly altered DCP (E) with some projections artifacts, and increased CC flow voids (F).

also of the inner retina [12]. Previous studies showed either thickening or thinning of inner retinal layers, and no consensus has been reached regarding the precise inner retinal changes occurring in RP yet [10, 12, 13]. It is likely to hypothesize that inner retinal involvement may vary as different phenotypic profiles of different RP subgroups. On the other side, all the studies agreed on correlating the inner retinal status with central retina function [10, 12–17]. Moreover, cystoid macular edema is a common structural OCT finding, occurring in approximately 10–50% of cases. The pathogenesis is still poorly understood; the current hypotheses include the breakdown of the inner blood-retinal barrier, the dysfunction of RPE pumps, the macular Müller cells impairment, possible autoimmune-related phenomena, and vitreomacular anomalies and traction [18, 19]. Other structural OCT-described findings include vitreoretinal interface alterations, epiretinal membrane, and macular hole [20]. Moreover, hyperreflective foci have been described in RP, correlating their number with the severity of the disease and the rate of progression [21, 22].

It is known that choroidal perfusion is impaired in RP; OCT-based imaging modalities may offer a detailed detection of choroidal features, improving the diagnostic workup of RP patients [23–26]. The choroid is not simply thinner than controls; a recent study highlighted how quantitative-based approaches can unveil specific RP choroidal patterns, characterized by different baseline features as well as the rate of progression. By combining the measure of choroidal thickness, Sattler layer thickness, Haller layer thickness, and choroidal vascularity index (CVI), it was possible to find three different RP choroidal patterns [27]. Pattern 1 is characterized by normal-appearing choroid, whereas Pattern 2 shows reduced Haller and Sattler layers. Moreover, Pattern 3 is characterized by reduced Haller and Sattler layers and choroidal caverns [27]. Pattern 1 was associated with better visual acuity and imaging parameters, and lower progression. Pattern 3 showed the worst baseline conditions and the fastest progression. Pattern 2 showed intermediate characteristics, since the morpho-functional status resulted worse than Pattern 1, although the 1-year progression resulted in unremarkable.

OCTA provided noninvasive evidence both of intraretinal and choroidal perfusion impairment in RP. Indeed, intraretinal vascular network impairment has been clearly shown by OCTA, together with degenerative changes occurring at the level of the choriocapillaris [28–31]. DCP represents the most altered plexus, as usually occurs almost in all retinal diseases. The main reason is related to the fact that DCP is a low-pressure network, thus earlier suffering from perfusion reductions associated with the disease-related pathological changes [1]. Hence, DCP alterations can be considered very sensitive to disease-related degenerative processes, although poorly specific. The use of quantitative OCTA metrics allowed us to distinguish two different RP vascular patterns, the first one characterized by better perfusion status and lower amount of vascular network disorganization, associated with lower progression and better visual outcome, than the second RP vascular pattern [32]. Vascular changes in RP occur as a consequence of progressive retinal homeostasis loss. However, the overall improvement of quantitative imaging techniques will allow us to better categorize different RP subtypes, also optimizing the diagnostic workup for future clinical trials.

3. Stargardt disease

STGD is one of the most common IRD associated with both recessive and dominant autosomal transmittance. Most of the patients show pathogenic variants of *ABCA4* gene, whose transmission is autosomal recessively inherited, while the remaining ones have autosomal dominant transmission mainly involving *PROM1* gene or *EVLOV4* [33–35]. The clinical presentation is usually characterized by bilateral central vision loss due to the macular involvement and fundoscopy-detectable

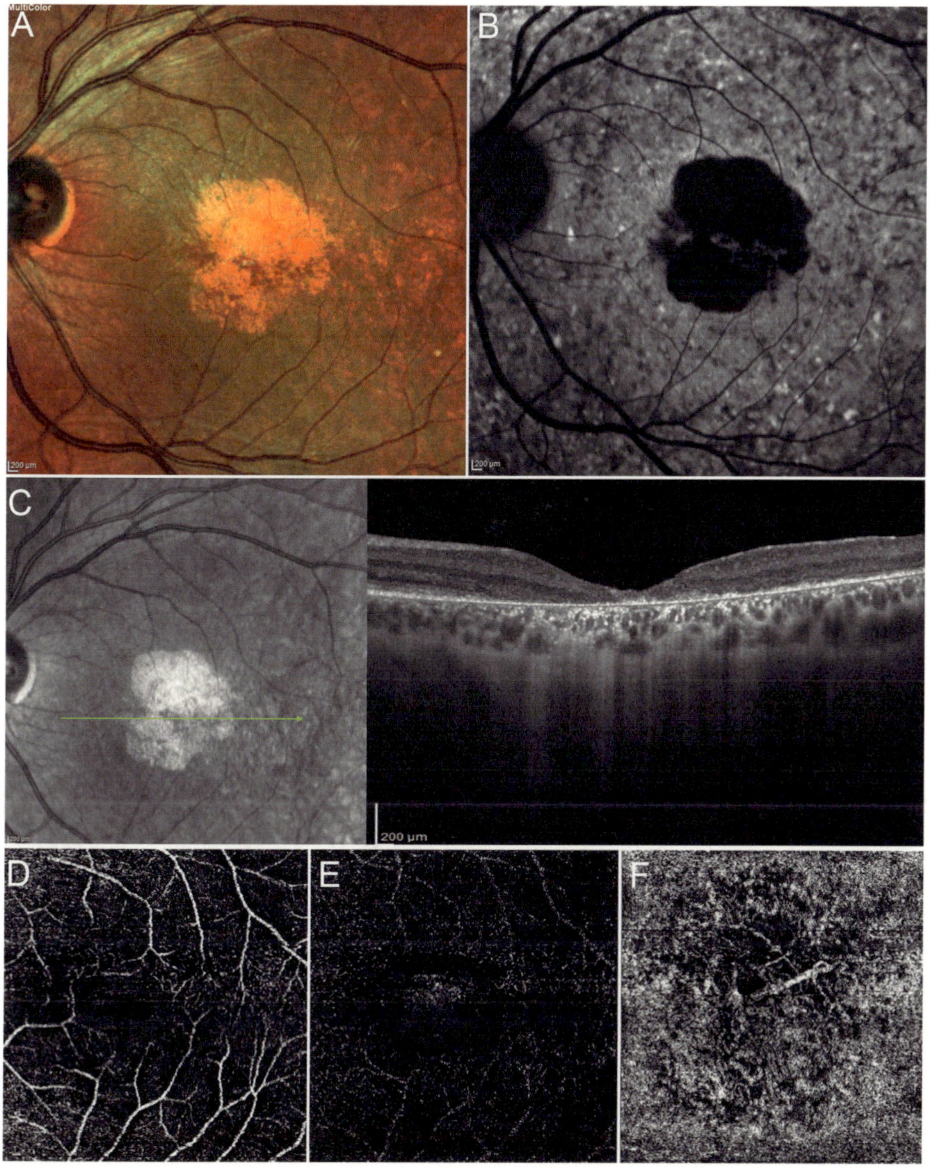

Figure 2.
Multimodal retinal imaging in STGD. Confocal multicolor image (A) shows hypopigmentation interesting the entire macular region. FAF image (B) confirms the presence of complete macular atrophy, with a thin line of partially preserved autofluorescent signal, together with sparse hyper- and hypoautofluorescence flecks over the entire posterior pole. Structural OCT (C) shows the complete disappearance of the central outer retinal bands, with choroidal hypertransmission and evident thinning of inner retinal layers. OCTA shows rarefied SCP (D), almost absent DCP (E) with some projections artifacts, and disappeared central CC with exposure of choroidal vessels, associated with markedly altered CC in the rest of the posterior pole (F).

flecks, namely sparse lipofuscin accumulations localized within the posterior pole and outside the vascular arcades. Age presentation follows two main peaks; the first is around 20 years of age with a more severe progression and worse prognosis, while the second one is around 40 years of age, typically presenting in a milder form [36]. A complete noninvasive multimodal retinal imaging STGD case is shown in **Figure 2**.

FAF examination is extremely useful in monitoring STGD progression by delineating atrophic regions, typically presenting as a central hypoautofluorescent area surrounded by a hyperautofluorescent ring [37, 38]. It is important to deeply assess two different sources of hypoautofluorescent signals. In particular, FAF can discriminate definitely decreased autofluorescence (DDAF), defined as a signal more than 90% black in Ref. to the optic nerve head, and questionably decreased autofluorescence (QDAF), defined as a signal included between 50% and 90% of reference black [39]. If DDAF corresponds to complete retinal atrophy, DDAF is more associated with the activity of the disease and the expansion of the atrophic margins. Near-infrared autofluorescence (NIR-AF) is a noninvasive modality focused on the assessment of melanin distribution. It is useful to describe the composition of flecks, which may disclose melanin content over lipofuscin, as well as to clearly detect the sparing of the fovea [40, 41]. If STGD has been mainly considered central dystrophy, the introduction of ultra-wide-field approaches expanded the knowledge regarding peripheral retinal involvement. In particular, different ultra-wide-field FAF patterns have been described, including Type I showing only central alterations without peripheral FAF changes; Type II is characterized by central atrophy and peripheral flecks; Type III presenting macular atrophy, peripheral FAF changes secondary to flecks, and progressively increasing extension of peripheral atrophy, further subclassified as IIIa, IIIb, and IIIc [42]. The peripheral extension of STGD-related alterations significantly correlated with the amount of central morpho-functional involvement, thus configurating completely different STGD phenotypes [43].

OCT is a mandatory investigation in STGD. Flecks are categorized into five different types (A, B, C, D, and E), based on their localization and their stage [44, 45]. In particular, Type A flecks resulted limited to the outer photoreceptors segment. Type B flecks showed protrusions through the interface of the inner photoreceptors segment. Type C flecks protrude up to the lower margin of the outer nuclear layer. Type D flecks lesions were characterized much more involved the thickness of the outer nuclear layer. Type E lesions appeared as drusen-like lesions. Structural OCT provides highly detailed pictures of the amount of outer and inner retinal degeneration, and of the number of hyperreflective foci [46–49]. The outer retinal bands are completely absent in the central part of the retina when atrophic changes occur, with typical choroidal hypertransmission. As previously described for RP, also in STGD it was possible to detect different clinically relevant choroidal patterns. In particular, Pattern 1 had a normal-appearing choroid, whereas Pattern 2 was characterized by alterations of Sattler or Haller choroidal layers. Pattern 3 showed significant alterations in both of the Sattler and Haller choroidal layers, whereas Pattern 4 was characterized by significant alterations in both of the Sattler and Haller choroidal layers and choroidal caverns [50]. The higher the choroidal pattern, the worse result of morpho-functional retinal status [50]. Moreover, choroidal patterns significantly correlated with the rate of STGD progression, resulting in the fastest in the Pattern 4 subtypes [50].

OCTA highlighted the significant vascular involvement of the intraretinal vascular network in STGD, showing a relationship between the amount of vascular impairment and both visual function, FAF, and structural OCT alterations [51–53]. In particular, DCP results highly altered already in early STGD stages, whereas the alterations at the level of the SCP occurs in later stages. The contribution of OCTA was improved by quantitative metrics segregating two different vascular patterns of STGD eyes [54]. Remarkably, the prevalence of foveal sparing was similar between the two OCTA subgroups, suggesting that the pathogenesis of foveal involvement might be even more complex, showing vascular supply impairment as a minor pathogenic element [54]. In addition, OCTA provided further support to the hypothesis of greater choriocapillaris involvement in STGD, compared with geographic atrophy secondary to age-related macular degeneration, providing the basis for a reliable differential diagnosis [55].

4. Best vitelliform macular dystrophy

Best vitelliform macular dystrophy (BVMD) is a rare IRD caused by dominant variants in the *BEST1* gene, encoding for the bestrophin-1 protein, a RPE chloride channel [56]. The typical clinical presentation is a central yellowish vitelliform or egg-yolk-like lesion, made by lipofuscin and photoreceptors' outer segment remnants [56]. The classic BVMD classification includes different stages. Stage I (subclinical) is characterized by the absence of biomicroscopic fundus abnormalities. Stage II (vitelliform) shows the typical egg yolk subretinal macular lesion. Stage III (pseudohypopyon) is characterized by partial fluid reabsorption in the upper part of the lesion and persistence of the yellowish subretinal deposition in the lower part. Stage IV (vitelliruptive) shows the reabsorption and breakdown of the material, giving a "scrambled egg" appearance. Stage V (atrophic/fibrotic) is complicated by the development of chorioretinal atrophy or macular neovascularization [57]. A complete noninvasive multimodal retinal imaging BVMD Stage IV case is shown in **Figure 3**.

FAF showed no alterations in the subclinical stage. Conversely, the vitelliform stage is characterized by a well-defined hyperautofluorescent alteration. The FAF signal progressively decreased passing through the pseudohypopyon stage, up to the vitelliruptive stage. Stage five is characterized by decreased FAF signal due to RPE atrophy [58]. However, BVMD-FAF appearance may be characterized by quite heterogeneous presentations, including classic, hyperautofluorescent, hypoautofluorescent, patchy, multifocal, and spoke-like patterns [59]. NIR-AF remarkably contributed to provide the pathognomonic sign of the subclinical BVMD stage, namely the presence of a central well-defined area of NIR-AF decrease [60]. The relationship between FAF assessment and retinal functionality is very close, making FAF a mandatory diagnostic tool for BVMD [61].

Regarding OCT findings, the subclinical stage may show only thickening of the interdigitation zone of cones and RPE in about 40% of cases [60]. The vitelliform stage is characterized by a dome-shaped subretinal hyperreflective lesion, which leaves space for the progressively increasing subretinal fluid hyporeflective signal occurring as pseudohypopyon and vitelliruptive stages proceed. The advanced stage shows either outer retinal atrophy or hyperreflective neovascular scar [62]. The presence of subretinal fluid is associated with worse visual acuity and retinal sensitivity values, compared with the persistence of vitelliform material [63–65]. Moreover, OCT was able to describe a clinically relevant outer retinal finding, namely the optically preserved islet in the context of the vitelliform accumulation, corresponding with EZ integrity and good macular function; its disappearance causes a remarkable decrease of visual acuity and retinal sensitivity [66, 67]. A high number of hyperreflective foci correlated with disease severity and progression rate also in BVMD [68]. Focal choroidal excavation is a frequent finding in BVMD, occurring in correspondence with a significant choroidal thinning [69, 70].

OCTA contributed by detecting a progressively increasing vascular impairment as the BVMD stages progress [71]. In the subclinical stage, OCTA was allowed to describe an early sign of choriocapillaris impairment, represented by central

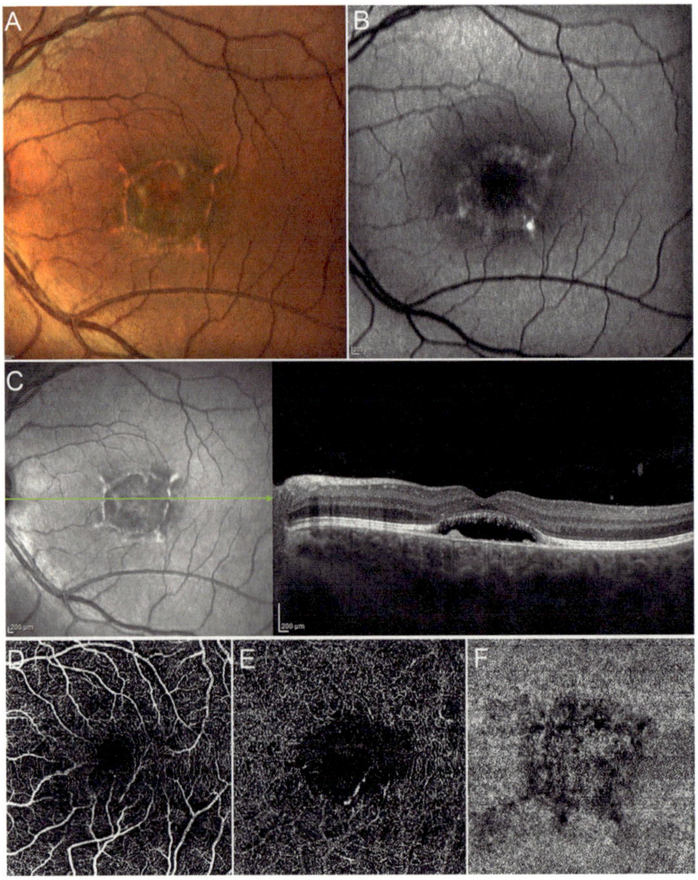

Figure 3.
Multimodal retinal imaging in BVMD. Confocal multicolor image (A) shows a scrumble egg appearance, which is suggestive of Stage IV vitelliruptive BVMD stage. FAF image (B) shows central alterations of the autofluorescent signal, either with hyper- or hypoautofluorescent changes. Structural OCT (C) shows the subretinal fluid corresponding with the vitelliform material in progressive reabsorption. OCTA shows almost preserved SCP (D), altered DCP with some alterations secondary to possible segmentation artifacts (E), and central CC alterations, probably related to the masking effect of the above localized subretinal fluid (F).

increased choriocapillaris flow voids [60]. In clinical stages, DCP first, followed by SCP, resulted altered in BVMD. However, the biggest OCTA contribution is regarding the radical change of macular neovascularization prevalence in BVMD. Indeed, before OCTA the prevalence of macular neovascularization was estimated at around 2–9% of cases [72]. After OCTA, the prevalence increases up to 65% of eyes [73, 74]. BVMD is characterized by two different macular neovascularization subtypes on OCTA: exudative and non-exudative. Exudative macular neovascularization is rare, more typical of Stages II and III, whereas non-exudative macular neovascularization develops very commonly in the advanced IV and V Stages [73]. Unfortunately, OCTA is less useful in evaluating the status of the choriocapillaris, since affected by the masking effect of the vitelliform material. Conversely, as expected, choriocapillaris is markedly impaired in advanced stages. Although the increased choriocapillaris flow voids detected in the subclinical stage may suggest that CC is effectively impaired in BVMD, further technological improvements are warranted to assess the choriocapillaris involvement in early BVMD stages.

5. Pigmented paravenous retinochoroidal atrophy

PPCRA is a rare chorioretinal atrophy characterized by perivenous aggregations of pigment clumps associated with peripapillary and radial zones of RPE atrophy following the course of retinal veins, usually bilateral and symmetric [75]. The etiopathogenesis of PPCRA is still unknown, and it is considered sporadic in most cases [76]. Patients are frequently asymptomatic, and the diagnosis is based on the typical fundus appearance. The natural history of the disease may be either nonprogressive or slowly progressive [75, 76]. In this chapter, we included PPCRA since many previous reports showed a familiar transmission of the disease, thus justifying the hypothesis of a genetic origin [77–82]. Interestingly, PPCRA has been also associated with pathogenic variants of *CRB1*

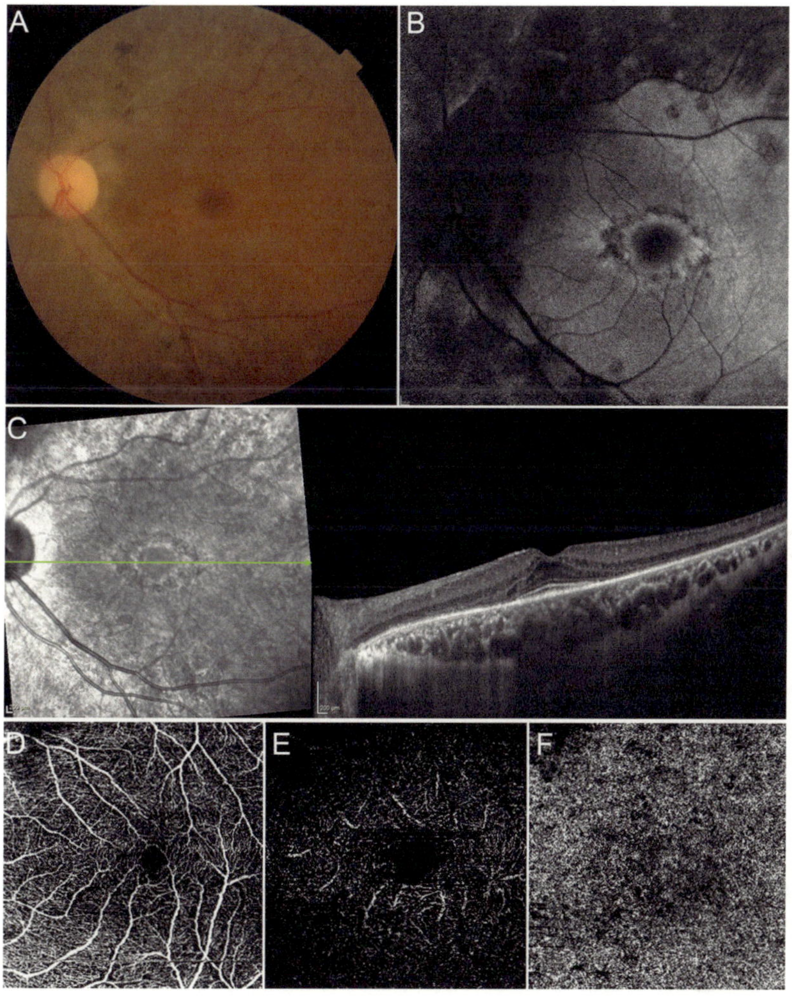

Figure 4.
Multimodal retinal imaging in PPCRA. Fundus image (A) shows evident hypopigmentation following the course of the vascular arcades, together with sparse alterations of the macular pigment. FAF image (B) confirms both the perivascular and the central alterations, detected as mainly hypoautofluorescent signals. Structural OCT (C) shows the disappearance of the peripheral outer retinal bands and some focal alterations localized at the level of the inner retina. OCTA shows almost preserved SCP (D), strongly altered DCP with many projection artifacts (E), and markedly altered CC (F).

gene [83]. The typical onset occurs between 10 and 67 years of age [84]. However, this time might be underestimated by the fact that PPCRA is usually asymptomatic, thus representing an incidental finding during routine ophthalmologic examinations. When present, the most common symptoms are mild visual loss, although visual acuity is usually preserved, reduction of the peripheral visual field and nyctalopia [84]. PPCRA has been classified into three categories based on the distribution of pigmentary changes: (I) "paravenous" type, distinguished by characteristic chorioretinal atrophy with pigment clumping that is geographically connected; (II) "focal" type, characterized by isolated chorioretinal atrophy with pigment clumping; (III) "confluent" type showing chorioretinal atrophy with diffuse bone spicules [76]. A complete noninvasive multimodal retinal imaging PPCRA case is shown in **Figure 4**.

FAF imaging is characterized by continuous hypoautofluorescent signal along the large retinal veins, surrounded by linear hyperautofluorescent signal extending to the periphery [76]. As expected, FAF alterations are different when considering the "paravenous", "focal", or "confluent" types.

OCT shows severe disruption of the RPE and outer retinal layers, usually associated with choroidal thinning, which may sometimes be the only pathological modification detected in PPCRA [76]. Moreover, OCTA may be normal in the early stages of the disease [85]. However, significant changes in deep capillary plexus and choriocapillaris have been recently described in a cohort of 12 patients affected by PPCRA [86]. The scientific interest in PPCRA is growing and noninvasive retinal imaging will undoubtedly provide clinically relevant data in the next future.

6. Pattern dystrophies

This paragraph is focused on pattern dystrophies in an attempt to offer a complete overview of OCT findings in IRD. However, in this case, the available literature is poor because of the rarity of these conditions, and in many cases, OCTA studies are completely absent.

Pattern dystrophies are a group of very rare autosomal dominant macular diseases characterized by very heterogeneous patterns of retinal pigment depositions and outer retinal alterations. Although a definite classification is still absent, pattern dystrophies are usually divided into five different categories: (I) Adult-onset foveomacular vitelliform dystrophy (AFVD); (II) Butterfly-shaped pigment dystrophy (BPD); (III) Reticular dystrophy; (IV) Multifocal Pattern Dystrophy Simulating Stargardt Disease (MPDSSD); and (V) Fundus pulverulentus [87]. However, especially looking at *PRPH2* gene variants, the clinical manifestations of pattern dystrophies may be extremely variable. In many cases, pattern dystrophies are caused by pathogenic variants of *PRPH2* gene, although other genes have been described as involved in the pathogenesis of these rare conditions. A complete noninvasive multimodal retinal imaging case diagnosed as pattern dystrophy associated with *PRPH2* gene variants is shown in **Figure 5**.

AFVD probably represents the most common pattern dystrophy, closely resembling BVMD, however is characterized by later onset, usually at 40–60 years of age. The clinical presentation is characterized by round, bilateral, symmetrical, grayish-yellow, lesions within the macular area. Visual acuity is usually preserved, and electrophysiology is within normal limits. Pathogenic variants are associated with *BEST1*, *PRPH2*, or *IMPG1* genes [88, 89]. FAF is characterized by hyperautofluorescent macular lesion in the vitelliform stage; changes in FAF signals follow the progressive degeneration of the outer retina. Structural OCT shows the presence of a subretinal

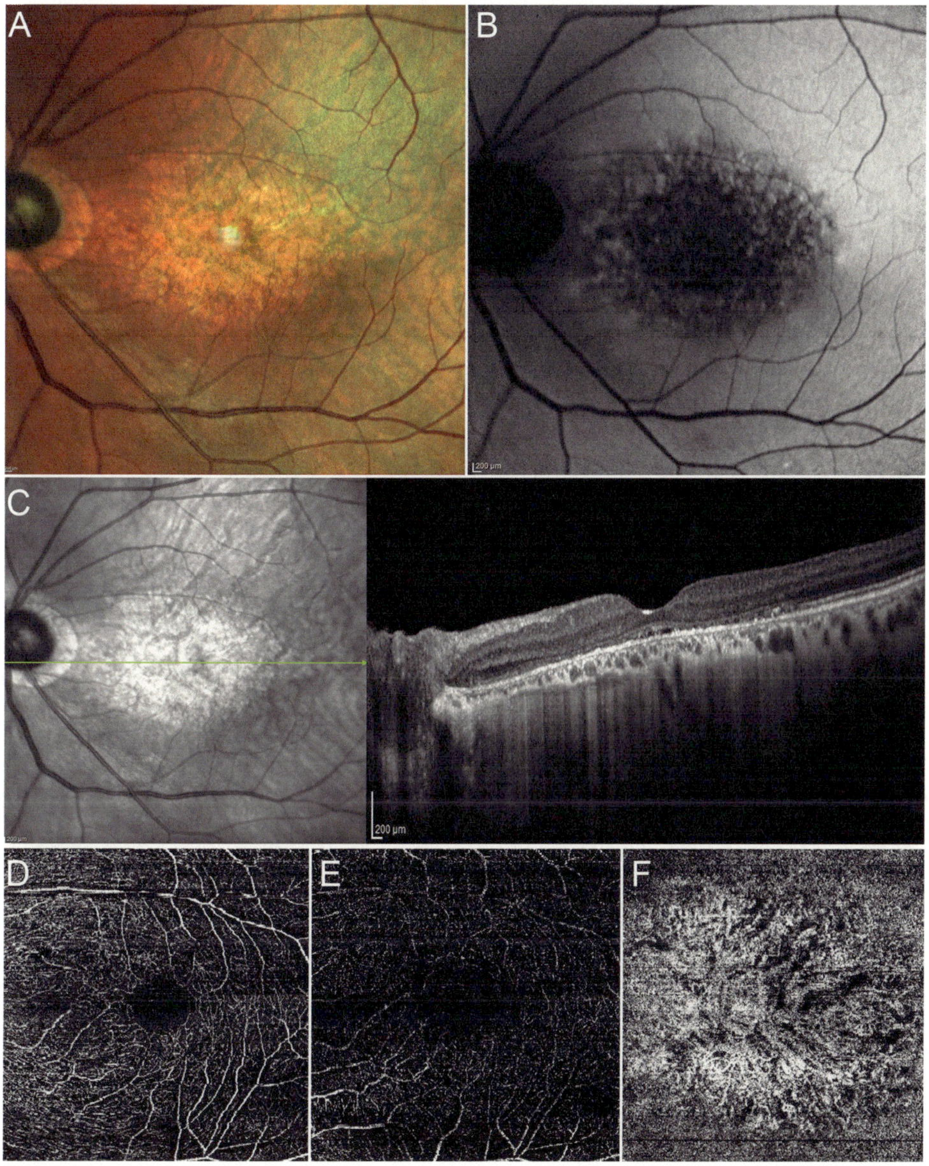

Figure 5.
Multimodal retinal imaging in PRPH2 gene-related pattern dystrophy. Confocal multicolor image (A) shows almost complete central retina atrophy. FAF image (B) confirms this finding, detecting a central mainly hypoautofluorescent signal. Structural OCT (C) shows disappeared or markedly attenuated outer retinal bands and inner retinal layers thinning. OCTA shows partially altered SCP with some segmentation and motion artifacts (D), strongly altered DCP with many projection artifacts (E), and absent central CC with exposure of choroidal vessels (F).

vitelliform lesion very similar to the vitelliform stage of BVMD. Vitelliruptive, as well as atrophic stages, can be detected also in AFVD. The clinical course of AFVD is usually more benign than BVMD. OCTA detects flow deficits especially interesting the DCP; neovascular complications can be well-reconstructed [90].

BPD has an onset around 20–40 years of age and is characterized by bilateral accumulation of yellowish or pigmented material in a butterfly wings-like pattern at the level of the RPE; visual acuity is usually good [91]. These butterfly-like pigment changes, corresponding both to hyper- and hypoautofluorescent signals on FAF, are well-detected on structural OCT, with heterogeneous patterns of outer retinal band alterations [92]. To the best of our knowledge, no OCTA studies are available for BPD.

Reticular dystrophy is characterized by a RPE network of hyperpigmentation, resembling a fishing net, extending from the macula in all directions, with sparing of the retinal periphery in early stages. In advanced stages, this network is complicated by atrophy [92, 93].

MPDSSD shows flecks-like alterations sparse within the entire posterior pole, with atrophic changes detected in the later stages of the disease. Flecks are often localized around the vascular arcades. Fundus appearance and OCT are very similar to STGD, and the differential diagnosis is mainly based on the detection of the autosomal dominant mechanism of inheritance [94].

Fundus pulverulentus is the rarest of all pattern dystrophies and is characterized by a granular appearance with coarse and punctiform mottling of the macular RPE. The clinical presentation is quite similar to age-related macular degeneration, leading to possible diagnostic delays [95]. Choroidal neovascularization has been described as a possible complication [96].

7. Final remarks

In this chapter, the most relevant OCT and OCTA findings in IRD have been described. Although several steps forward have been performed, especially looking at the most frequent IRD types, further prospective studies are needed to provide a definite categorization of each IRD and to improve the knowledge regarding the pathogenesis and the patterns of progression. Moreover, it should always be taken into account that OCT and OCTA are prone to imaging artifacts. These can be categorized as patient-related, technology-related, and disease-related artifacts [1]. Patient-related artifacts are mainly related to patients' fixation and collaboration, leading to many artifacts, including motion and blinking artifacts. Technology-related artifacts are related to the current limitation of the post-processing algorithm in carefully segmenting images and detecting signals, thus leading to biases, such as projection and segmentation artifacts. Disease-related artifacts are secondary to the disease-related alterations affecting the retinal structures, potentially masking or altering the detection of the signals. In brief, the higher are both fixation instability and pathological modifications of retinal structures, the higher will be the artifacts affecting the quality and the interpretation of OCT and OCTA images. This is particularly true for IRD, since in most of the cases, the retinal structures are remarkably impaired, and the visual function of the patients is strongly compromised. For these reasons, from one side both expert and nonexpert ophthalmologists should be familiar with imaging artifacts, to avoid misinterpretation of the findings. On the other end, further technological improvements are warranted to make noninvasive retinal imaging even more reliable for performing the diagnostic workup of IRD patients.

8. Conclusions

In conclusion, we provided an updated overview regarding the retinal imaging characteristics of RP, STGD, BVMD, and PPCRA, highlighting how heterogeneous can be the clinical spectrum and how useful the contribution of OCT and OCTA diagnostic techniques. Moreover, we provided a brief updated description of current imaging findings in pattern dystrophies. The advances in knowledge regarding the above-described as well as all the other IRD are mandatory to reach the high level of information required to develop useful treatments. In addition, the proper use of imaging techniques is fundamental to optimize the selection of patients for potential clinical trials, allowing the categorization of clinically different diseases' subgroups, and for the monitoring of treatments' effect on the course of the disease. Moreover, the even larger employment of artificial intelligence-based diagnostic approaches will undoubtedly benefit from the improvements of quantitative multimodal retinal imaging approaches, which are able to provide a very high amount of detailed, objective, and easily reproducible data. However, especially looking at very rare IRD types, further studies are warranted to collect more cases and to provide more data regarding the imaging characteristics of these diseases. The future of IRD management is promising, and noninvasive retinal imaging technologies will further contribute to improve the ophthalmologic diagnostic workup and, consequently, the quality of life of IRD patients.

Financial disclosures

Francesco Bandello consultant for: Alcon (Fort Worth, Texas, USA), Alimera Sciences (Alpharetta, Georgia, USA), Allergan Inc. (Irvine, California, USA), Farmila-Thea (Clermont-Ferrand, France), Bayer Shering-Pharma (Berlin, Germany), Bausch And Lomb (Rochester, New York, USA), Genentech (San Francisco, California, USA), Hoffmann-La-Roche (Basel, Switzerland), NovagaliPharma (Évry, France), Novartis (Basel, Switzerland), Sanofi-Aventis (Paris, France), Thrombogenics (Heverlee, Belgium), Zeiss (Dublin, USA). All other authors have no relevant disclosures to declare.

Author details

Alessandro Arrigo*, Lorenzo Bianco, Alessio Antropoli, Andrea Saladino, Alessandro Berni, Maurizio Battaglia Parodi and Francesco Bandello
IRCCS San Raffaele Scientific Institute, Vita-Salute San Raffaele University, Milan, Italy

*Address all correspondence to: alessandro.arrigo@hotmail.com

References

[1] Arrigo A, Aragona E, Battaglia Parodi M, Bandello F. Quantitative approaches in multimodal fundus imaging: State of the art and future perspectives. Progress in Retinal and Eye Research. 2022;**2022**:101111. DOI: 10.1016/j.preteyeres.2022.101111

[2] Amato A, Arrigo A, Aragona E, Manitto MP, Saladino A, Bandello F, et al. Gene therapy in inherited retinal diseases: An update on current state of the art. Frontier Medicine (Lausanne). 2021;**8**:750586. DOI: 10.3389/fmed.2021.750586

[3] Hartong DT, Berson EL, Dryja TP. Retinitis pigmentosa. Lancet. 2006;**368**(9549):1795-1809. DOI: 10.1016/S0140-6736(06)69740-7

[4] Robson AG, El-Amir A, Bailey C, Egan CA, Fitzke FW, Webster AR, et al. Pattern ERG correlates of abnormal fundus autofluorescence in patients with retinitis pigmentosa and normal visual acuity. Investigative Ophthalmology & Visual Science. 2003;**44**(8):3544-3550. DOI: 10.1167/iovs.02-1278

[5] Robson AG, Tufail A, Fitzke F, Bird AC, Moore AT, Holder GE, et al. Serial imaging and structure-function correlates of high-density rings of fundus autofluorescence in retinitis pigmentosa. Retina. 2011;**31**(8):1670-1679. DOI: 10.1097/IAE.0b013e318206d155

[6] Sujirakul T, Lin MK, Duong J, Wei Y, Lopez-Pintado S, Tsang SH. Multimodal imaging of central retinal disease progression in a 2-year mean follow-up of retinitis pigmentosa. American Journal of Ophthalmology. 2015;**160**(4):786-98.e4. DOI: 10.1016/j.ajo.2015.06.032

[7] Battaglia Parodi M, La Spina C, Triolo G, Riccieri F, Pierro L, Gagliardi M, et al. Correlation of SD-OCT findings and visual function in patients with retinitis pigmentosa. Graefe's Archive for Clinical and Experimental Ophthalmology. 2016;**254**(7):1275-1279. DOI: 10.1007/s00417-015-3185-x

[8] Rangaswamy NV, Patel HM, Locke KG, Hood DC, Birch DG. A comparison of visual field sensitivity to photoreceptor thickness in retinitis pigmentosa. Investigative Ophthalmology & Visual Science. 2010;**51**(8):4213-4219. DOI: 10.1167/iovs.09-4945

[9] Wen Y, Klein M, Hood DC, Birch DG. Relationships among multifocal Electroretinogram amplitude, visual field sensitivity, and SD-OCT receptor layer thicknesses in patients with retinitis pigmentosa. Investigative Ophthalmology & Visual Science. 2012;**53**(2):833-840. DOI: 10.1167/iovs.11-8410

[10] Liu G, Liu X, Li H, Du Q, Wang F. Optical coherence tomographic analysis of retina in retinitis pigmentosa patients. Ophthalmic Research. 2016;**56**(3):111-122. DOI: 10.1159/000445063

[11] Arrigo A, Aragona E, Battaglia O, Saladino A, Amato A, Borghesan F, et al. Outer retinal tubulation formation and clinical course of advanced age-related macular degeneration. Scientific Reports. 2021;**11**(1):14735. DOI: 10.1038/s41598-021-94310-5

[12] Aleman TS, Cideciyan AV, Sumaroka A, Schwartz SB, Roman AJ, Windsor EA, et al. Inner retinal abnormalities in X-linked retinitis pigmentosa with RPGR mutations. Investigative Ophthalmology & Visual Science. 2007;**48**(10):4759-4765. DOI: 10.1167/iovs.07-0453

[13] Hood DC, Lin CE, Lazow MA, Locke KG, Zhang X, Birch DG. Thickness of receptor and post-receptor retinal layers in patients with retinitis pigmentosa measured with frequency-domain optical coherence tomography. Investigative Ophthalmology & Visual Science. 2009;**50**(5):2328-2336. DOI: 10.1167/iovs.08-2936

[14] Jones BW, Pfeiffer RL, Ferrell WD, Watt CB, Marmor M, Marc RE. Retinal remodeling in human retinitis pigmentosa. Experimental Eye Research. 2016;**150**:149-165. DOI: 10.1016/j.exer.2016.03.018

[15] Funatsu J, Murakami Y, Nakatake S, Akiyama M, Fujiwara K, Shimokawa S, et al. Direct comparison of retinal structure and function in retinitis pigmentosa by co-registering microperimetry and optical coherence tomography. PLoS One. 2019;**14**(12):e0226097. DOI: 10.1371/journal.pone.0226097

[16] Hara A, Nakazawa M, Saito M, Suzuki Y. The qualitative assessment of optical coherence tomography and the central retinal sensitivity in patients with retinitis pigmentosa. PLoS One. 2020;**15**(5):e0232700. DOI: 10.1371/journal.pone.0232700

[17] Arrigo A, Aragona E, Perra C, Saladino A, Amato A, Bianco L, et al. Morphological and functional involvement of the inner retina in retinitis pigmentosa. Eye (Lond). 29 Jun 2022. DOI: 10.1038/s41433-022-02139-7. Epub ahead of print

[18] Hajali M, Fishman GA, Anderson RJ. The prevalence of cystoid macular oedema in retinitis pigmentosa patients determined by optical coherence tomography. The British Journal of Ophthalmology. 2008;**92**(8):1065-1068. DOI: 10.1136/bjo.2008.138560

[19] Strong S, Liew G, Michaelides M. Retinitis pigmentosa-associated cystoid macular oedema: Pathogenesis and avenues of intervention. The British Journal of Ophthalmology. 2017;**101**(1):31-37. DOI: 10.1136/bjophthalmol-2016-309376

[20] Testa F, Rossi S, Colucci R, Gallo B, Di Iorio V, della Corte M, Azzolini C, Melillo P, Simonelli F. Macular abnormalities in Italian patients with retinitis pigmentosa. The British Journal of Ophthalmology. 2014;**98**(7):946-950. DOI: 10.1136/bjophthalmol-2013-304082

[21] Kuroda M, Hirami Y, Hata M, Mandai M, Takahashi M, Kurimoto Y. Intraretinal hyperreflective foci on spectral-domain optical coherence tomographic images of patients with retinitis pigmentosa. Clinical Ophthalmology Auckland NZ. 2014;**8**:435-440. DOI: 10.2147/OPTH.S58164

[22] Nagasaka Y, Ito Y, Ueno S, Terasaki H. Number of Hyperreflective foci in the outer retina correlates with inflammation and photoreceptor degeneration in retinitis Pigmentosa. Ophthalmological Retina. 2018;**2**(7):726-734. DOI: 10.1016/j.oret.2017.07.020

[23] Langham ME, Kramer T. Decreased choroidal blood flow associated with retinitis pigmentosa. Eye. 1990;**4**(Pt 2):374-381. DOI: 10.1038/eye.1990.50

[24] Ayton LN, Guymer RH, Luu CD. Choroidal thickness profiles in retinitis pigmentosa. Clinical & Experimental Ophthalmology. 2013;**41**(4):396-403. DOI: 10.1111/j.1442-9071.2012.02867.x

[25] Falsini B, Anselmi GM, Marangoni D, D'Esposito F, Fadda A, Di Renzo A, et al. Subfoveal choroidal blood flow and central retinal function

in retinitis pigmentosa. Investigative Ophthalmology & Visual Science. 2011;**52**(2):1064-1069. DOI: 10.1167/iovs.10-5964

[26] Mrejen S, Spaide RF. Optical coherence tomography: Imaging of the choroid and beyond. Survey of Ophthalmology. 2013;**58**(5):387-429. DOI: 10.1016/j.survophthal.2012.12.001

[27] Arrigo A, Bordato A, Romano F, Aragona E, Grazioli A, Bandello F, et al. Choroidal patterns in retinitis Pigmentosa: Correlation with visual acuity and disease progression. Translational Vision Science & Technology. 2020;**9**(4):17. DOI: 10.1167/tvst.9.4.17

[28] Ling L, Gao F, Zhang Q, He T, Zhao Y, Xing Y, et al. Optical coherence tomography angiography assessed retinal and choroidal microvasculature features in patients with retinitis pigmentosa: A meta-analysis. BioMed Research International. 2019;**2019**:6723917. DOI: 10.1155/2019/6723917

[29] Liu R, Lu J, Liu Q, Wang Y, Cao D, Wang J, et al. Effect of choroidal vessel density on the ellipsoid zone and visual function in retinitis Pigmentosa using optical coherence tomography angiography. Investigative Ophthalmology & Visual Science. 2019;**60**(13):4328-4335. DOI: 10.1167/iovs.18-24921

[30] Battaglia Parodi M, Cicinelli MV, Rabiolo A, Pierro L, Gagliardi M, Bolognesi G, et al. Vessel density analysis in patients with retinitis pigmentosa by means of optical coherence tomography angiography. The British Journal of Ophthalmology. 2017;**101**(4):428-432. DOI: 10.1136/bjophthalmol-2016-308925

[31] Hagag AM, Wang J, Lu K, Harman G, Weleber RG, Huang D, et al. Projection-resolved optical coherence tomographic angiography of retinal plexuses in retinitis pigmentosa. American Journal of Ophthalmology. 2019;**204**:70-79. DOI: 10.1016/j.ajo.2019.02.034

[32] Arrigo A, Romano F, Albertini G, Aragona E, Bandello F, Battaglia PM. Vascular patterns in retinitis pigmentosa on swept-source optical coherence tomography angiography. Journal of Clinical Medicine. 2019;**8**(9):1425. DOI: 10.3390/jcm8091425

[33] Heath Jeffery RC, Mukhtar SA, McAllister IL, Morgan WH, Mackey DA, Chen FK. Inherited retinal diseases are the most common cause of blindness in the working-age population in Australia. Ophthalmic Genetics. 2021;**42**(4):431-439. DOI: 10.1080/13816810.2021.1913610

[34] Lu LJ, Liu J, Adelman RA. Novel therapeutics for Stargardt disease. Graefe's Archive for Clinical and Experimental Ophthalmology. 2017;**255**(6):1057-1062. DOI: 10.1007/S00417-017-3619-8

[35] Lee W, Xie Y, Zernant J, Yuan B, Bearelly S, Tsang SH, et al. Complex inheritance of ABCA4 disease: Four mutations in a family with multiple macular phenotypes. Human Genetics. 2016;**135**(1):9-19. DOI: 10.1007/S00439-015-1605-Y

[36] Collison FT, Fishman GA. Visual acuity in patients with Stargardt disease after age 40. Retina. 2018;**38**(12):2387-2394. DOI: 10.1097/IAE.0000000000001903

[37] Lois N, Halfyard AS, Bird AC, Holder GE, Fitzke FW. Fundus autofluorescence in stargardt macular dystrophy-fundus flavimaculatus. American Journal of Ophthalmology.

2004;**138**(1):55-63. DOI: 10.1016/j.ajo.2004.02.056

[38] Zhao PY, Abalem MF, Nadelman D, et al. Peripheral pigmented retinal lesions in Stargardt disease. American Journal of Ophthalmology. 2018;**188**:104-110. DOI: 10.1016/J.AJO.2017.12.011

[39] Ervin AM, Strauss RW, Ahmed MI, Birch D, Cheetham J, Ferris FL 3rd, et al. A workshop on measuring the progression of atrophy secondary to Stargardt disease in the ProgStar studies: Findings and lessons learned. Translational Vision Science and Technology. 2019;**8**(2):16. DOI: 10.1167/tvst.8.2.16

[40] Gomes NL, Greenstein VC, Carlson JN, Tsang SH, Smith RT, Carr RE, et al. A comparison of fundus autofluorescence and retinal structure in patients with Stargardt disease. Investigative Ophthalmology & Visual Science. 2009;**50**(8):3953-3959. DOI: 10.1167/IOVS.08-2657

[41] Jauregui R, Nuzbrokh Y, Su PY, Zernant J, Allikmets R, Tsang SH, et al. Retinal pigment epithelium atrophy in recessive Stargardt disease as measured by short-wavelength and near-infrared autofluorescence. Translational Vision Science & Technology. 2021;**10**(1):1-11. DOI: 10.1167/TVST.10.1.3

[42] Klufas MA, Tsui I, Sadda SR, Hosseini H, Schwartz SD. Ultrawidefield autofluoresence in ABCA4 Stargardt disease. Retina. 2018;**38**(2):403-415. DOI: 10.1097/IAE.0000000000001567

[43] Arrigo A, Grazioli A, Romano F, Aragona E, Marchese A, Bordato A, et al. Multimodal evaluation of central and peripheral alterations in Stargardt disease: A pilot study. The British Journal of Ophthalmology. 2020;**104**(9): 1234-1238. DOI: 10.1136/bjophthalmol-2019-315148

[44] Rotenstreich Y, Fishman GA, Anderson RJ. Visual acuity loss and clinical observations in a large series of patients with Stargardt disease. Ophthalmology. 2003;**110**(6):1151-1158. DOI: 10.1016/S0161-6420(03)00333-6

[45] Voigt M, Querques G, Atmani K, Leveziel N, Massamba N, Puche N, et al. Analysis of retinal flecks in fundus flavimaculatus using high-definition spectral-domain optical coherence tomography. American Journal of Ophthalmology. 2010;**150**(3):330-337. DOI: 10.1016/J.AJO.2010.04.001

[46] Berisha F, Feke GT, Aliyeva S, Hirai K, Pfeiffer N, Hirose T. Evaluation of macular abnormalities in Stargardt's disease using optical coherence tomography and scanning laser ophthalmoscope microperimetry. Graefe's Archive for Clinical and Experimental Ophthalmology. 2009;**247**(3):303-309. DOI: 10.1007/S00417-008-0963-8

[47] Khan KN, Kasilian M, Mahroo OAR, Tanna P, Kalitzeos A, Robson AG, et al. Early patterns of macular degeneration in ABCA4-associated retinopathy. Ophthalmology. 2018;**125**(5):735-746. DOI: 10.1016/J.OPHTHA.2017.11.020

[48] Lee W, Nõupuu K, Oll M, Duncker T, Burke T, Zernant J, et al. The external limiting membrane in early-onset Stargardt disease. Investigative Ophthalmology & Visual Science. 2014;**55**(10):6139-6149. DOI: 10.1167/IOVS.14-15126

[49] Battaglia Parodi M, Sacconi R, Romano F, Bandello F. Hyperreflective foci in Stargardt disease: 1-year follow-up. Graefe's Archive for Clinical and Experimental Ophthalmology. 2019;**257**(1):41-48. DOI: 10.1007/S00417-018-4167-6

[50] Arrigo A, Grazioli A, Romano F, Aragona E, Bordato A, di Nunzio C, et al.

Choroidal patterns in Stargardt disease: Correlations with visual acuity and disease progression. Journal of Clinical Medicine. 2019;**8**(9):1388. DOI: 10.3390/jcm8091388

[51] Battaglia Parodi M, Cicinelli MV, Rabiolo A, Pierro L, Bolognesi G, Bandello F. Vascular abnormalities in patients with Stargardt disease assessed with optical coherence tomography angiography. The British Journal of Ophthalmology. 2017;**101**(6):780-785. DOI: 10.1136/bjophthalmol-2016-308869

[52] Mastropasqua R, Toto L, Borrelli E, Di Antonio L, Mattei PA, Senatore A, et al. Optical coherence tomography angiography findings in Stargardt disease. PLoS One. 2017;**12**(2):e0170343. DOI: 10.1371/journal.pone.0170343

[53] Guduru A, Lupidi M, Gupta A, Jalali S, Chhablani J. Comparative analysis of autofluorescence and OCT angiography in Stargardt disease. The British Journal of Ophthalmology. 2018;**102**(9):1204-1207. DOI: 10.1136/bjophthalmol-2017-311000

[54] Arrigo A, Romano F, Aragona E, di Nunzio C, Sperti A, Bandello F, et al. OCTA-based identification of different vascular patterns in Stargardt disease. Translational Vision Science & Technology. 2019;**8**(6):26. DOI: 10.1167/tvst.8.6.26

[55] Müller PL, Pfau M, Möller PT, Nadal J, Schmid M, Lindner M, et al. Choroidal flow signal in late-onset Stargardt disease and age-related macular degeneration: An OCT-Angiography Study. Investigative Ophthalmology & Visual Science. 2018;**59**(4):AMD122-AMD131. DOI: 10.1167/iovs.18-23819

[56] Boon CJ, Klevering BJ, Leroy BP, Hoyng CB, Keunen JE, den Hollander AI. The spectrum of ocular phenotypes caused by mutations in the BEST1 gene. Progress in Retinal and Eye Research. 2009;**28**(3):187-205. DOI: 10.1016/j.preteyeres.2009.04.002

[57] Gass JDM. Best's disease. In: Stereoscopic Atlas of Macular Diseases. Diagnosis and Treatment. St Louis, MO: Mosby; 1997

[58] Lima de Carvalho JR, Jr PM, Chen L, Chiang J, Tsang SH, Sparrow JR. Multimodal imaging in Best vitelliform macular dystrophy. Investigative Ophthalmology & Visual Science. 2019;**60**(6):2012-2022. DOI: 10.1167/iovs.19-26571

[59] Parodi MB, Iacono P, Campa C, Del Turco C, Bandello F. Fundus autofluorescence patterns in Best vitelliform macular dystrophy. American Journal of Ophthalmology. 2014;**158**(5):1086-1092. DOI: 10.1016/j.ajo.2014.07.026

[60] Parodi MB, Arrigo A, Calamuneri A, Aragona E, Bandello F. Multimodal imaging in subclinical Best vitelliform macular dystrophy. The British Journal of Ophthalmology. 2022;**106**(4):564-567. DOI: 10.1136/bjophthalmol-2020-317635

[61] Parodi MB, Iacono P, Del Turco C, Triolo G, Bandello F. Functional assessment of the fundus autofluorescence pattern in Best vitelliform macular dystrophy. Graefe's Archive for Clinical and Experimental Ophthalmology. 2016;**254**(7):1297-1302. DOI: 10.1007/s00417-015-3194-9

[62] Battaglia Parodi M, Iacono P, Romano F, Bolognesi G, Fasce F, Bandello F. Optical coherence tomography in Best vitelliform macular dystrophy. European Journal of Ophthalmology. 2017;**27**(2):201-204. DOI: 10.5301/ejo.5000878

[63] Battaglia Parodi M, Iacono P, Romano F, Bandello F. Spectral domain optical coherence tomography features in different stages of Best vitelliform macular dystrophy. Retina. 2018;**38**(5):1041-1046. DOI: 10.1097/IAE.0000000000001634

[64] Battaglia Parodi M, Castellino N, Iacono P, Chowers I, Empeslidis T, Goldstein M, et al. Microperimetry in Best vitelliform macular dystrophy. Retina. 2018;**38**:841-848

[65] Battaglia Parodi M, Bianco L, Arrigo A, Saladino A, Antropoli A, Pina A, et al. Clinical correlation between optical coherence tomography biomarkers and retinal sensitivity in Best Vitelliform macular dystrophy. Translational Vision Science & Technology. 2022;**11**(9):24. DOI: 10.1167/tvst.11.9.24

[66] Romano F, Arrigo A, Leone PP, Saladino A, Bandello F, Battaglia PM. Altered ellipsoid zone reflectivity and deep capillary plexus rarefaction correlate with progression in Best disease. The British Journal of Ophthalmology. 2020;**104**(4):461-465. DOI: 10.1136/bjophthalmol-2019-313980

[67] Romano F, Arrigo A, Leone PP, Bandello F, Battaglia PM. Short-term modifications of ellipsoid zone in Best Vitelliform macular dystrophy. Retina. 2021;**41**:1010-1017. DOI: 10.1097/IAE.0000000000002977

[68] Parodi MB, Romano F, Sacconi R, Casati S, Marchini G, Bandello F, et al. Intraretinal hyperreflective foci in Best vitelliform macular dystrophy. Retina. 2018;**38**(12):2379-2386. DOI: 10.1097/IAE.0000000000001893

[69] Battaglia Parodi M, Casalino G, Iacono P, Introini U, Adamyan T, Bandello F. The expanding clinical spectrum of choroidal excavation in macular dystrophies. Retina. 2018;**38**(10):2030-2034. DOI: 10.1097/IAE.0000000000001805

[70] Battaglia Parodi M, Sacconi R, Iacono P, Del Turco C, Bandello F. Choroidal thickness in Best vitelliform macular dystrophy. Retina. 2016;**36**(4):764-769. DOI: 10.1097/IAE.0000000000000759

[71] Battaglia Parodi M, Romano F, Cicinelli MV, Rabiolo A, Arrigo A, Pierro L, et al. Retinal vascular impairment in Best vitelliform macular dystrophy assessed by means of optical coherence tomography angiography. American Journal of Ophthalmology. 2018;**187**:61-70. DOI: 10.1016/j.ajo.2017.12.013

[72] Clemett R. Vitelliform dystrophy: Long-term observations on New Zealand pedigrees. Australian and New Zealand Journal of Ophthalmology. 1991;**19**:221-227. DOI: 10.1111/j.1442-9071.1991.tb00665.x

[73] Parodi MB, Arrigo A, Bandello F. Optical coherence tomography angiography quantitative assessment of macular neovascularization in Best vitelliform macular dystrophy. Investigative Ophthalmology & Visual Science. 2020;**61**(6):61. DOI: 10.1167/iovs.61.6.61

[74] Guduru A, Gupta A, Tyagi M, Jalali S, Chhablani J. Optical coherence tomography angiography characterisation of Best disease and associated choroidal neovascularisation. The British Journal of Ophthalmology. 2018;**102**(4):444-447. DOI: 10.1136/bjophthalmol-2017-310586

[75] Lee EK, Lee SY, Oh BL, Yoon CK, Park UC, Yu HG. Pigmented Paravenous Chorioretinal atrophy: Clinical Spectrum

and multimodal imaging characteristics. American Journal of Ophthalmology. 2021;**224**:120-132. DOI: 10.1016/j.ajo.2020.12.010

[76] Huang HB, Zhang YX. Pigmented paravenous retinochoroidal atrophy (review). Experimental and Therapeutic Medicine. 2014;**7**(6):1439-1445. DOI: 10.3892/etm.2014.1648

[77] Traboulsi EI, Maumenee IH. Hereditary pigmented paravenous chorioretinal atrophy. Archives of Ophthalmology. 1986;**104**(11):1636-1640. DOI: 10.1001/archopht.1986.01050230074036

[78] Noble KG. Hereditary pigmented paravenous chorioretinal atrophy. American Journal of Ophthalmology. 1989;**108**(4):365-369. DOI: 10.1016/s0002-9394(14)73302-1

[79] Bozkurt N, Bavbek T, Kazokoğlu H. Hereditary pigmented paravenous chorioretinal atrophy. Ophthalmic Genetics. 1998;**19**(2):99-104. DOI: 10.1076/opge.19.2.99.2317

[80] Small KW, Anderson WB Jr. Pigmented paravenous retinochoroidal atrophy. Discordant expression in monozygotic twins. Archives of Ophthalmology. 1991;**109**(10):1408-1410. DOI: 10.1001/archopht.1991.01080100088048

[81] Obata R, Yanagi Y, Iriyama A, Tamaki Y. A familial case of pigmented paravenous retinochoroidal atrophy with asymmetrical fundus manifestations. Graefe's Archive for Clinical and Experimental Ophthalmology. 2006;**244**(7):874-877. DOI: 10.1007/s00417-005-0179-0

[82] Al-Husainy S, Sarodia U, Deane JS. Pigmented paravenous retinochoroidal atrophy: Evidence of progression to macular involvement in a family with a 42-year history. Eye (London, England). 2001;**15**(Pt 3):329-330. DOI: 10.1038/eye.2001.105

[83] McKay GJ, Clarke S, Davis JA, Simpson DA, Silvestri G. Pigmented paravenous chorioretinal atrophy is associated with a mutation within the crumbs homolog 1 (CRB1) gene. Investigative Ophthalmology & Visual Science. 2005;**46**(1):322-328. DOI: 10.1167/iovs.04-0734

[84] Shona OA, Islam F, Robson AG, Webster AR, Moore AT, Michaelides M. Pigmented paravenous chorioretinal atrophy: Detailed clinical study of a large cohort. Retina. 2019;**39**(3):514-529. DOI: 10.1097/IAE.0000000000001950

[85] Ranjan R, Jain MA, Verghese S, Manayath GJ, Narendran V. Multimodal imaging of pigmented paravenous retinochoroidal atrophy. European Journal of Ophthalmology. 2022;**32**(1):NP125-NP129. DOI: 10.1177/1120672120965489

[86] Battaglia Parodi M, Arrigo A, Chowers I, Jarc-Vidmar M, Shpigel M, Bandello F, et al. Optical coherence tomography angiography findings in pigmented paravenous chorioretinal atrophy. Retina. 2022;**42**(5):915-922. DOI: 10.1097/IAE.0000000000003407

[87] Gass JMD. Stereoscopic Atlas of Macular Disease. Philadelphia, PA: Elsevier; 1997

[88] Renner AB, Tillack H, Kraus H, Kohl S, Wissinger B, Mohr N, et al. Morphology and functional characteristics in adult vitelliform macular dystrophy. Retina. 2004;**24**(6):929-939. DOI: 10.1097/00006982-200412000-00014

[89] Arnold JJ, Sarks JP, Killingsworth MC, Kettle EK, Sarks SH. Adult vitelliform macular degeneration:

A clinicopathological study. Eye (London, England). 2003;**17**(6):717-726. DOI: 10.1038/sj.eye.6700460

[90] Joshi KM, Nesper PL, Fawzi AA, Mirza RG. Optical coherence tomography angiography in adult-onset foveomacular vitelliform dystrophy. Retina. 2018;**38**(3):600-605. DOI: 10.1097/IAE.0000000000001565

[91] Deutman AF, van Blommestein JD, Henkes HE, Waardenburg PJ, Solleveld-van DE. Butterfly-shaped pigment dystrophy of the fovea. Archives of Ophthalmology. 1970;**83**(5):558-569. DOI: 10.1001/archopht.1970.00990030558006

[92] Boon CJ, den Hollander AI, Hoyng CB, Cremers FP, Klevering BJ, Keunen JE. The spectrum of retinal dystrophies caused by mutations in the peripherin/RDS gene. Progress in Retinal and Eye Research. 2008;**27**(2):213-235. DOI: 10.1016/j.preteyeres.2008.01.002

[93] Marano F, Deutman AF, Pinckers AJ, Aandekerk AL, Rijneveld WJ. Reticular dystrophy of the retinal pigment epithelium and choroidal neovascularization. A fluorescein and ICGV study. Acta Ophthalmologica Scandinavica. 1997;**75**(1):22-27. DOI: 10.1111/j.1600-0420.1997.tb00243.x

[94] Boon CJ, van Schooneveld MJ, den Hollander AI, van Lith-Verhoeven JJ, Zonneveld-Vrieling MN, Theelen T, et al. Mutations in the peripherin/RDS gene are an important cause of multifocal pattern dystrophy simulating STGD1/fundus flavimaculatus. The British Journal of Ophthalmology. 2007;**91**(11):1504-1511. DOI: 10.1136/bjo.2007.115659

[95] Pinckers A. Patterned dystrophies of the retinal pigment epithelium: A review. Ophthalmic Paediatrics and Genetics. 1988;**9**(2):77-114. DOI: 10.3109/13816818809031483

[96] Battaglia PM. Choroidal neovascularization in fundus pulverulentus. Acta Ophthalmologica Scandinavica. 2002;**80**(5):559-560. DOI: 10.1034/j.1600-0420.2002.800521.x

Chapter 4

Optical Coherence Tomography in Retinopathy of Prematurity

Artemiy Kokhanov, Ye He, Pooja Nikki Bisarya and Irena Tsui

Abstract

Retinopathy of prematurity (ROP) is a disease that uniquely affects prematurely born infants. This disease is caused by disordered retinal vascular proliferation and may lead to blindness. The gold standard for ROP screening, diagnosis and monitoring is indirect ophthalmoscopy examination. Optical coherence tomography (OCT) has recently been used in ROP affected infants and children in research settings. It has provided further understanding of retinal vascular development and visualization of subtle subclinical features that otherwise go undetected. In school-aged children, OCT has become an essential tool for monitoring macular sequelae of ROP such as retained inner retinal layers, epiretinal membrane, subretinal fluid, and retinoschisis. This chapter reviews the current use of OCT in infants with ROP as well as older children with history of ROP.

Keywords: cystoid macular edema, foveal avascular zone, optical coherence tomography, plus disease, prematurity, retinal detachment, retinopathy of prematurity, retinoschisis

1. Introduction

Retinopathy of prematurity (ROP) is a disorder unique to prematurely born neonates. It stems from abnormal retinal vascular proliferation which may lead to permanent damage to the retina and retinal detachment. It remains to be the main cause of childhood blindness throughout the world notwithstanding the major progress in management [1]. The first description of ROP came in 1942 by Terry [2]. At the time the condition was called retrolental fibroplasia and was thought to represent persistent fetal vasculature related to prematurity [2]. Afterwards it was determined that those findings were not innate, but rather developed postnatally in response to exogenous factors, such as exposure to oxygen [3]. Judicial use of supplemental oxygen led to reduction in incidence of ROP [4]. The advancements in neonatal care and increased survival of very low and extremely low birth weight neonates in developed countries resulted in the "second wave' of ROP [5]. The "third wave" came with the recent rapid expansion of neonatal services in developing countries where control of complications of preterm birth is lagging [6]. Each year about 32,300 prematurity survivors worldwide are impacted by permanent vision impairment due to ROP [7]. In recent years, with the increased use of OCT, there has been an ever-increasing interest in using optical coherence tomography (OCT) to comprehend ocular development as well as to detect long term macular sequelae of ROP [8]. In this chapter the utilization of OCT in infants and children with ROP will be discussed.

2. Early uses and challenges of neonatal OCT

Adoption of OCT into neonatal population has been limited due to various reasons such as absence of available equipment for quick and accurate imaging without sedation [9]. Early attempts to use OCT in neonatal population were made in operating room under general anesthesia [10, 11]. Vinekar et al. were among the first to use handheld OCT in premature infants. Using the handheld device that was made from a tabletop spectral domain OCT scanner they showed clinically undetected abnormal findings of cystoid spaces and greater foveal thickness in patients with stage 2 ROP. Also, they demonstrated the possibility of OCT imaging of unanesthetized infants at bedside [12].

3. Imaging technique

While utilization of modified unmounted tabletop OCT scanners has been reported in literature, this is challenging due to the limited portability of the device [11, 13]. Commercially available portable handheld and arm-mounted OCT systems made it feasible to obtain imaging in premature infants, but at this time they are still not widely used in clinical practice [14, 15].

The eye of a premature infant and the adult eye have many structural and optical dissimilarities. The axial length of the premature eye undergoes precipitant growth during neonatal period and then slows progressively afterwards. The cornea has steeper curvature in neonates compared to adults [15, 16]. Refractive error pattern switches from slight myopia in neonatal period towards slight hyperopia in infancy. In addition, newborn eyes have greater astigmatism [15]. If these features are not taken into consideration, difficulties, such as poor image clarity and clipping artifacts can be encountered. Thereby, imaging protocols must be configured to account for these age-specific properties [17]. OCT systems with shorter acquisition times such as spectral domain (SD) and swept source (SS) are faster making them more suitable for infants [9]. OCT angiography (OCT-A) is a rather new quick and non-invasive imaging technique to perform visualization and quantitative analysis of retinal vasculature as well as the evaluation of retinal blood flow without the need for an intravenous or intravitreal injection of a contrast agent [18–20]. This provides an alternative to fluorescein angiography. OCT-A can be used to generate various foveal vascular characteristics including vessel perfusion density, vessel length density and vascular diameter index [21]. A limitation of OCT/OCT-A is that they do not easily capture the peripheral retina where stages of ROP occur.

The imaging can be done with minimal to no discomfort to the patient. A speculum is generally needed [20, 22]. Oral sucrose may be given to comfort the patient. Arm mounted imaging systems may greatly facilitate the task as there would be no need to support the weight of the scanner. A second person would operate the software and capture the images [17, 22]. Ocular lubrication should be applied before imaging to create a stable tear film for clearer images. Scleral depression may be used to manipulate the eye position and improve peripheral views [23]. Ultimately, it has been reported that OCT imaging may even be less stressful than indirect ophthalmoscopy examinations that are routinely done to evaluate for ROP [24]. Implementation of age-specific techniques was evaluated by Maldonado et al. and it was found that the average time per imaging session decreased and there was no significant change of vital signs from baseline [15].

4. OCT findings in neonatal ROP

The standard for ROP screening has been the eye examination using an indirect ophthalmoscope. OCT allowed to visualize structures and characteristics that have been previously clinically unnoticed. Among those are preretinal tissue, epiretinal membrane, shallower foveal depression, presence of distinct inner retinal layers at the foveal center, macular edema, retinoschisis, retinal detachment, changes associated with plus disease, and optic nerve changes. Occult findings that can be visualized by OCT imaging might play a considerable role in the vision abnormalities in children with history of ROP. OCT findings have the potential to be used as an adjunct for ROP screening and monitoring. Widefield imaging using swept source OCT combined with scleral depression has the capability to visualize peripheral retinal pathology. This may have the ability to allow objective quantitative evaluation of the ROP classification. The components of ROP classification can be measured more discreetly with the use of OCT compared to indirect ophthalmoscopy [25]. In the future, it might be achievable to segment the peripheral vascular-avascular junction, create objective cutoffs for ROP stages and quantify plus disease with more objectivity using artificial intelligence derived metrics [26].

4.1 Preretinal tissue

The exact histopathologic makeup of preretinal tissue is not precisely known, but it is thought to represent remnants of hyaloidal vasculature or small isolated lumps of neovascular tissue overlying the retina [27]. These lesions also have been referred to as popcorn retinopathy [28]. It has been previously reported that the presence of popcorn retinopathy increases the risk of disease progression as well as the development of plus disease and requirement for laser photocoagulation [28]. The ability to monitor the preretinal tissue may be of importance in disease surveillance.

4.2 Epiretinal membrane

Epiretinal membrane comprises a layer of cellular proliferation on the inner surface of the retina. Epiretinal membranes are frequently seen in premature neonates [17]. Lee et al. reported that epiretinal membranes were present in 32% of cases evaluated for ROP while. They were detected by OCT imaging while not seen on indirect ophthalmoscopy examination. In nearly a third of the patients the epiretinal membrane generation foveal deformation with loss of the fovea depression [29]. The association was made between epiretinal membrane and the development of vitreous bands suggesting a tractional pathogenesis of this finding in the affected infants [20, 30]. Nonetheless, the exact clinical significance of epiretinal membrane in premature infants with ROP remains unknown, and more studies are needed to evaluate its value.

4.3 Immature retinal and choroidal morphology

Overall inner retina layer thickness at the foveal center decreases and outer retinal thickness at foveal center increases over time in the preterm period, which is driven by centrifugal and centripetal displacement of inner and outer retinal cells, respectively.

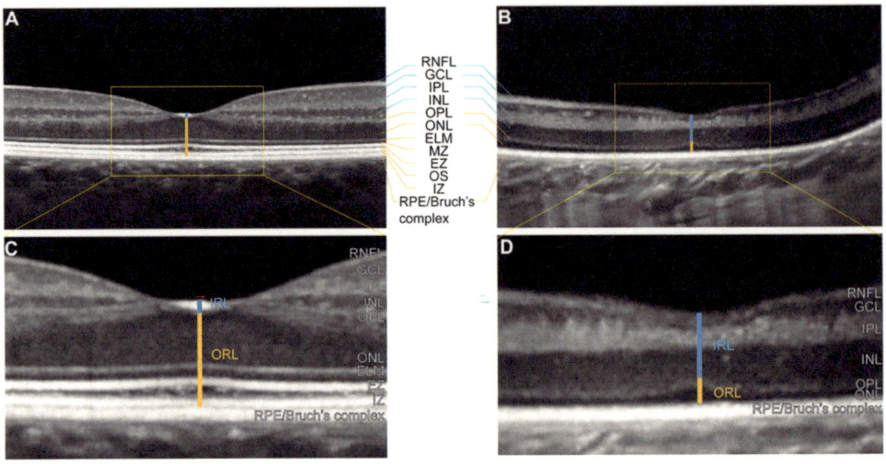

Figure 1.
Differences of foveal OCT B-scan in the healthy adult and developing retina. (A, C) Foveal OCT B-scan image from a 24-year-old adult born at term age. (B, D) Foveal OCT B-scan image from a 34-week postmenstrual age (PMA) infant (born at 25 weeks GA, birth weight 605 g). From top to bottom, the retinal layers are: Retinal nerve fiber layer (RNFL), ganglion cell layer (GCL), inner plexiform layer (IPL), inner nuclear layer (INL), outer plexiform layer (OPL), outer nuclear layer (ONL), external limiting membrane (ELM), myoid zone of photoreceptors (MZ), ellipsoid zone of photoreceptors (EZ), outer segments of photoreceptors (OS), interdigitation zone (IZ), and retinal pigment epithelium (RPE)/Bruch's complex. Inner retinal layers (IRL) are indicated by the blue vertical line. Outer retinal layers (ORL) are indicated by the orange vertical line. Note that the ELM, MZ, EZ, and IZ are not apparent in the immature developing retina (B, D). Adapted from [31] with permission.

It has been reported that compared to term born infant, premature infant or ROP infant eyes usually has shallower foveal pit, retain inner retinal layers at foveal center, thinner outer retinal layers, and indistinctive external limiting membrane band and ellipsoid zone (**Figure 1**) [32–34].

Choroid is another component of the eye that could be impacted in premature or ROP infancy. It has been reported that several factors including gestational age, ROP status, pulmonary status and oxygen supplementation may affect choroidal thickness [8, 22, 35, 36]. However, the impact of changes in choroidal thickness on long-term visual outcomes is still under investigation.

4.4 Retinoschisis

Retinoschisis, or abnormal splitting or retina's neurosensory layers, is not common in ROP. However, the incidence of it is not known for the most part due to the relative difficulty on indirect ophthalmoscopy or digital eye imaging systems. Some features commonly encountered in premature infants, such as corneal haze, presence of tunica vasculosa lentis or vitreous hemorrhage make particularly difficult [37].

4.5 Retinal detachment

In spite of treatment efforts, a number of prematurely born infants develop advanced ROP with retinal detachment. Accurate detection of retinal detachment is crucial in decision making process as well as in predicting future vision outcomes.

Differentiation of retinoschisis from retinal detachment and determination of foveal involvement can be a difficult task. Likewise, the decision whether to intervene may be a great challenge. OCT has been shown the ability to assess the exact location of detachment, assess the degree of retinal elevation, estimate foveal involvement and distinguish retinal detachment from retinoschisis [10, 38–40]. Shallow retinal detachments that are not seen on indirect ophthalmoscopy also can be detected earlier on OCT imaging [41]. Detecting post-laser photocoagulation exudative retinal detachment using OCT has been reported as well [42].

4.6 Plus disease

Plus disease is defined as increased venous dilatation and arteriolar tortuosity of the posterior retinal vessels in at least two quadrants [43]. It is an important clinical sign of ROP used to identify patients that require treatment. OCT can provide further objective understanding of structural changes that occur in plus disease. Three-dimensional reconstruction of OCT images can allow visualization of vessel tortuosity not only in two dimensions, but in the third dimension across the retinal depth as well [17]. Special OCT views such as Retinal Vessel Shadow View have been proposed for evaluation of plus disease [44]. Furthermore, OCT may detect vessel elevation, a feature that is known to be related to ROP severity [45].

With the aim of reducing the impact of individual OCT features and to ensure a more comprehensive evaluation of vascular changes, a Vascular Abnormality Score on OCT (VASO) was suggested (**Table 1**). In this scoring system more uncommon features are more heavily weighted. Thus, uncommon findings have more impact on VASO score. A cut-off value of 2 was proposed. Subjects in the plus disease group had significantly higher VASO than scores in the control group. The mean difference in VASO score was larger when imaging was performed before 37 weeks corrected gestational age [45].

4.7 Macular edema

Macular edema has been a subject of recent research thanks to the ease of its detection by OCT (**Figure 2**). This is a feature that is usually not detected by traditional

Optical coherence tomography characteristics	Points
Vessel elevation	
Mild	1
Severe	2
Scalloped retinal layers	
Involving IPL	1
Involving OPL	2
Hyporeflective vessels	2
Retinal spaces	2

Table 1.
Vascular abnormality score on optical coherence tomography (VASO).

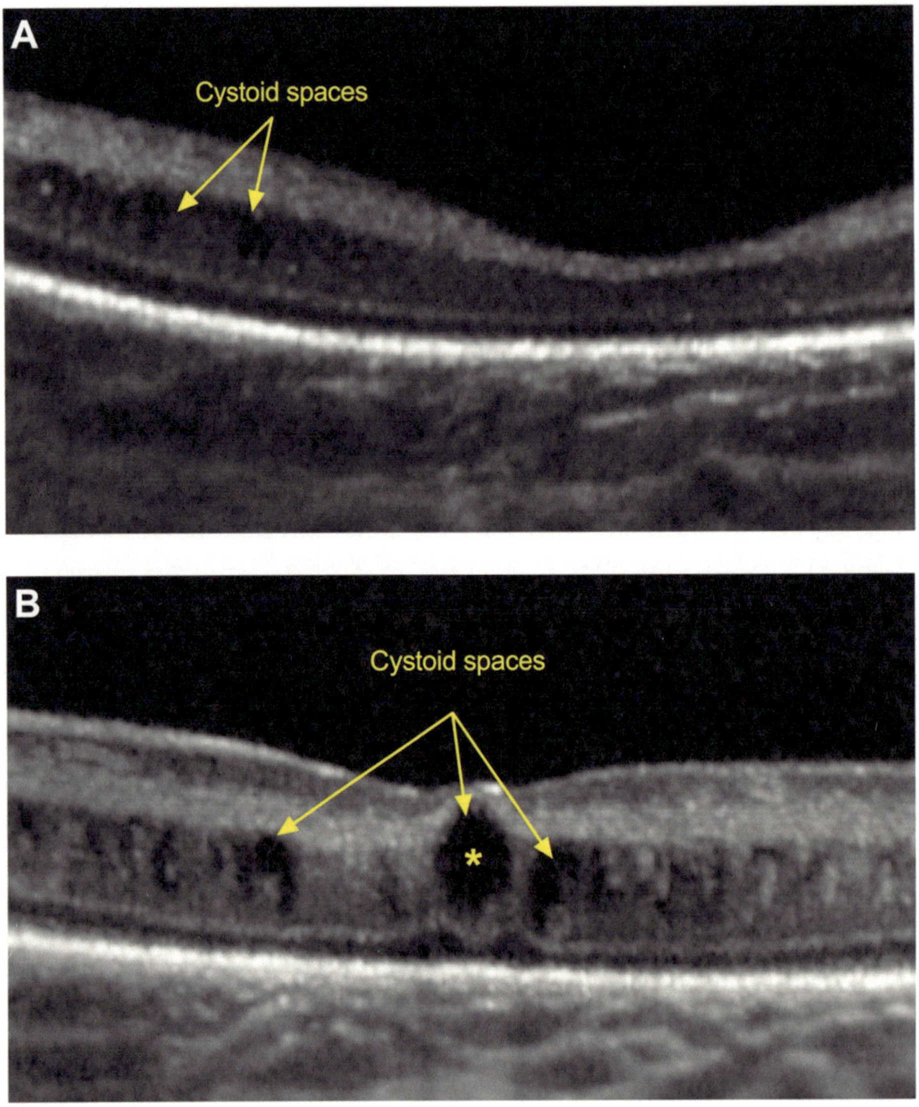

Figure 2.
Macular edema. Foveal OCT B-scan image in an eye of a preterm infant born at 28 weeks gestational age (birth weight 1220 g) imaged at 32 weeks postmenstrual age. Macular edema was only observed in the inner nuclear layer at the parafovea (A). Foveal OCT B-scan image in an eye of a preterm infant born at 25 weeks gestational age (birth weight 605 g) imaged at 42 weeks postmenstrual age. Macular edema was also only observed in the inner nuclear layer but at both fovea and parafovea (B). Yellow asterisk is located at within a cystoid space at fovea.

indirect ophthalmoscopy, and it often remains undiagnosed during infancy. Different studies use different nomenclature for this feature, which include "retinal cystoid structures" [29], "foveal/macular changes" [12], "cystoid macular changes" [46] and "macular edema of prematurity" (MEOP). This phenomenon frequently resolves spontaneously [17]. Maldonado et al. found cystoid macular edema (CME) in 50% of premature neonates imaged between 31 and 36 weeks of corrected gestational age. CME persisted in all subjects through 36 weeks of corrected gestational age. The study was not designed for long term follow up, however the resolution of CME was observed in 9 out of 17 subjects after 37 weeks corrected gestational age [47]. Vinekar et al. performed a study on 74 patients and CME was found in 16% of patients. The resolution was reported in 100% of patients imaged at 52 weeks of corrected gestational age [12].

CME seen in premature infants is different than CME seen in adult patients. Thus, in premature infants CME is located exclusively in inner nuclear layer while in adults cystoid structures may be found in multiple retinal layers [47, 48]. Adult CME is caused by both extracellular accumulation of fluid as well as intracellular swelling of Muller cells whereas infantile CME may be represented principally by the swelling of Muller cells, or potentially extracellular fluid accumulation that is bridged by Muller cells [47, 49].

The exact etiology of CME encountered in premature infants is not precisely known. Several hypotheses have been suggested. Maldonado et al. and Vinekar et al. have proposed that CME develops as a result of the effects of neurohumoral factors, primarily vascular endothelial growth factor (VEGF). Edema may be attributed to increased vascular permeability that is caused by increased concentration of VEGF [12, 47]. This theory is plausible given the role of VEGF in the pathogenesis of ROP. Among 27 different cytokines measured in the vitreous body VEGF was found to be of the highest concentrations in patients with advanced ROP compared to controls [50]. Nevertheless, it was observed that CME might develop after intravitreal injection of bevacizumab, a VEGF inhibitor [46]. This led to a thought that other pathogenetic factors, such as mechanical traction exerted on the macula, might be involved. Tractional pathogenesis theory is also supported by an association of CME with the development of vitreous bands [30]. Furthermore, Erol et al. have suggested that lower retina pigment epithelium cell density might promote the development of CME [51].

As noted earlier, CME is a common finding in premature neonates, and its mere presence may not be necessarily associated with ROP. It may represent a non-pathologic transient stage of foveal development. Currently, there is no consensus whether the severity of CME is correlated with ROP. Dubis et al. reported in their study that severity of CME does not appear to be correlated with ROP stage [46]. However, greater severity of CME as evidenced by increased central foveal thickness, inner nuclear layer and fovea-to-parafoveal thickness ratio has been found by Maldonado et al. to be linked with higher ROP stage, presence of plus disease and the need for laser photocoagulation [47]. Similarly, Erol et al. reported that frequency and severity of CME go up with increasing ROP stage [51]. As the retinal changes have been found to correlate with gestational age and birth weight, it still continues to be unclear if those findings are due to preterm birth alone or are in connection with the effects of ROP and its management [52]. Other concomitant systemic factors may influence the development of CME. Among these factors are hypo- and hyperoxia, acidosis, arterial hypotension, presence of hemodynamically significant patent ductus arteriosus, infection, intraventricular hemorrhage, necrotizing enterocolitis, transfusion of blood products and apnea of prematurity [46]. However, Maldonado et al. made an attempt to correlate some of these factors (specifically Apgar scores at 1 and 5 minutes of life, PDA ligation, culture-proven sepsis, surgical necrotizing enterocolitis, presence of intraventricular hemorrhage, periventricular leukomalacia, bronchopulmonary dysplasia, and hydrocephalus) with CME and could not establish the association [47].

Anwar et al. reported in their study a correlation between foveal width and retinopathy of prematurity. The foveal width was increasing in the ROP group and decreasing in the non-ROP group. This difference of trajectory was found to be independent of gestational age and birth weight – variables that are certainly concurrent with the extent of prematurity. This difference was more apparent particularly at earlier corrected gestational age. This phenomenon has the potential to be of utility when differentiating between premature infants that need further ROP screening from those that do not. Also, it has the potential to be used as a predictor of ROP that requires treatment [53].

Another possible association that might be of interest is the correlation of CME with neurodevelopmental outcomes in prematurely born children. Rothman et al. studied neurodevelopmental outcomes in 53 very preterm infants at 18 to 24 corrected gestational age. Infants who had CME detected during routine ROP screening eye examinations were found to have poorer language and motor skills on Bayley Scales for Infant and Toddler development when compared to the infants who did not have CME [54]. Thereby, detection and evaluation of CME using OCT imaging have the potential to serve as the predictor of neurodevelopmental outcomes in prematurely born infants.

4.8 Optic nerve changes

Previously, the understanding of optic nerve development originated from different histopathology experiments [55]. The appearance of OCT has allowed for in-vivo studies of the optic nerve in humans. OCT has been used broadly for optic nerve evaluation in adults, however the use of it for infant optic nerve assessment has been limited until now. Preterm infants who underwent ROP screening were found to have larger vertical cup diameter and cup-to-disc ratio than their term counterparts in a pilot study of 44 preterm and 52 term infants. These parameters were found to have a weak association with neurologic pathology such as periventricular leukomalacia, and lower cognitive Bayley scores [56]. However, future larger prospective studies are needed before definite conclusions can be made.

5. OCT in children with history of ROP

OCT has been studied for assessment of premature children beyond the neonatal period and infancy as well. The impact of prematurity itself, ROP and ROP treatment have been studied. Features that were observed during infancy also persist in childhood and throughout adolescence, these include shallow foveal pit (**Figures 3–5**),

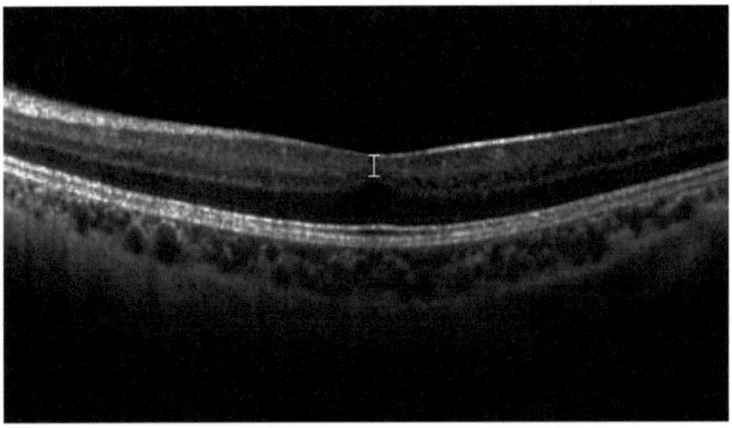

Figure 3.
Abnormal foveal contour in a premature-born child. Foveal OCT B-scan in an eye of a 12 years old premature-born child with shallow foveal pit and retain inner retinal layers at foveal center (yellow vertical line).

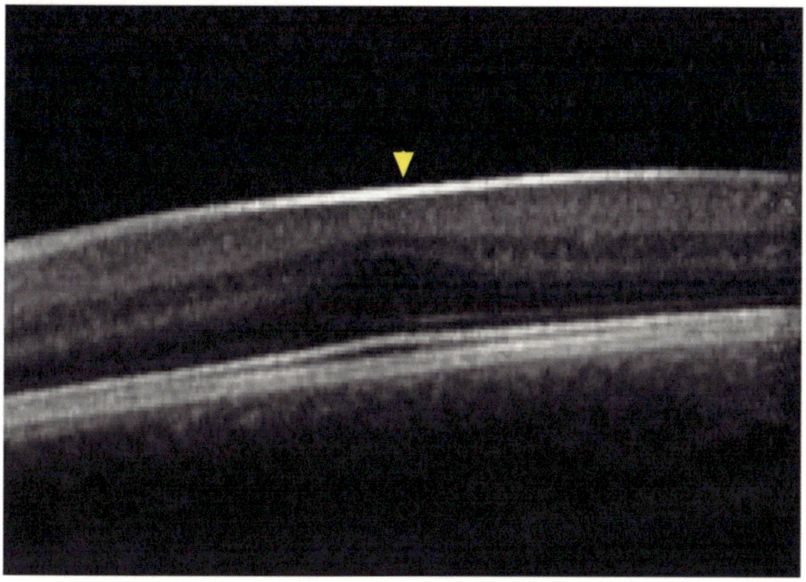

Figure 4.
Epiretinal membrane (ERM). Foveal OCT cross-sectional B-scan in an eye of a 10 years old premature-born child. ERM is presented as hyperreflective layer (yellow arrowhead) overlaying on the retina.

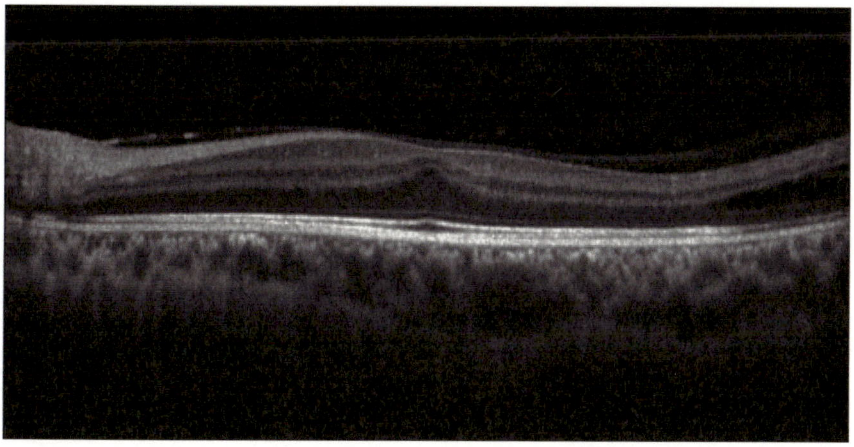

Figure 5.
OCT images demonstrating examples of retinoschisis. OCT B-scan image of temporal retinoschisis in a 17-year-old with history of ROP without treatment. Note the macular anomalies including blunting or shallow of the foveal depression and the presence of the inner retina at the foveal center.

remain inner retinal layers at foveal center (**Figures 3–5**), ERM (**Figure 4**), retinoschisis (**Figure 5**), and Optic nerve changes (**Figure 6**).

OCT findings demonstrated that total thickness of the retina is increased in premature children with and without ROP compared with their term counterparts [57, 58]. Tariq et al. reported increased thickness of the central macula and thinning of the outer macula in prematurely born teenagers when compared to those born at term [59].

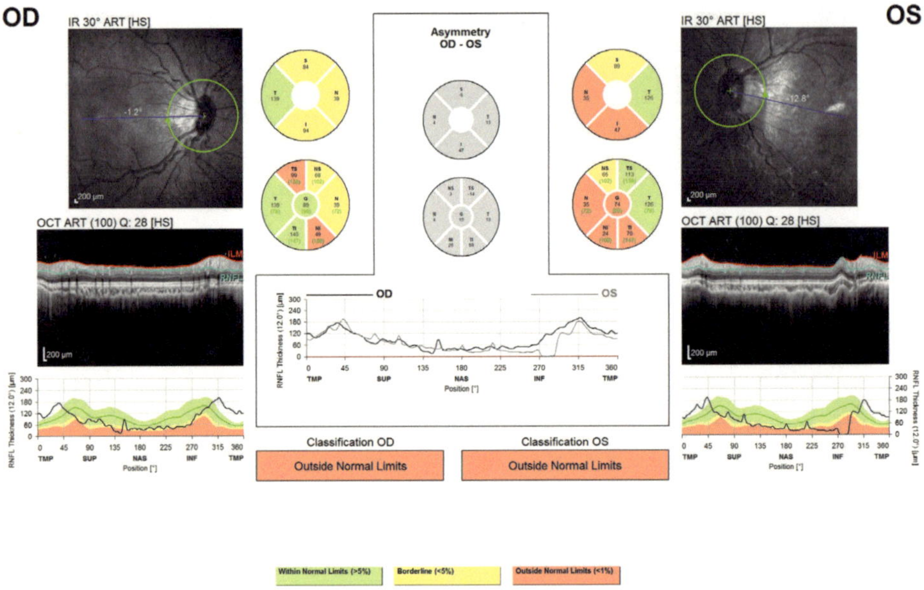

Figure 6.
Optic nerve atrophy.

Foveal avascular zone (FAZ) is a landmark that has been studied broadly in the recent years. It was found to be remarkably reduced or absent in children children with a history of prematurity with or without ROP [57, 60]. Smaller avascular zone presumably denotes arrest of normal development of retinal neurovasculature induced by premature birth [21, 61]. Positive correlation has been described between FAZ and gestational age and birth weight [62]. At the same time, FAZ was found to be smaller in children with history of treated ROP compared with those with history of spontaneously regressed ROP [21, 57]. However, the former group of patients had lower gestational age and birth weight. As such, the described differences in FAZ might be induced by more significantly immature vasculature at the time of birth [57]. Regarding vessel density, studies have reported that children with a history of prematurity have higher vessel density at the fovea when compared to healthy children [63–65], while other studies did not reveal a difference in vessel density [21, 66, 67].

Children that were born prematurely have been shown to have significantly smaller choroidal thickness 3.0 mm temporal to the fovea than children born at term. Though, choroidal thickness in other locations did not significantly differ. ROP stage had marginally significant inverse correlation with choroidal thickness 3.0 mm temporal to the fovea [68].

Children who were subject to laser treatment of ROP have been shown to have significantly narrower anterior chamber angle (ACA) compared to prematurely born children not treated with laser. In its turn, the ACA was correlated with the degree of myopia. Given the lack of statistically significant difference between ACA in preterm controls versus term controls, it can be assumed that laser treatment and not gestational age contributes to the narrow ACA [60].

Another finding reported in children with history of ROP is increased disc-to-fovea ratio, which can be detected by OCT. This finding may be caused by foveal dragging which in turn is a consequence of cicatricial ROP. However, this association needs to be evaluated further in studies with larger cohorts [69].

6. Conclusion

OCT has been an important tool used for diagnosis and management of various ophthalmic conditions in adults and older children. Its use in neonates and infants has been limited to research. OCT has demonstrated its utility in expanding and supplying the new knowledge of infant ocular morphology and providing new insights into the pathophysiology of ROP. Also, it has provided the new outlook for retinal vascular development and allowed for a three-dimensional view of pathological ROP findings. In addition, OCT has allowed for visualization of subclinical findings that are not evident on conventional clinical examination. Thereby, OCT has the potential to become an indispensable addition to conventional binocular indirect ophthalmoscopy screening for ROP. It is feasible that OCT will aid in early identification of ROP that is at higher risk of poor outcomes and allow for timely intervention. Currently, many morphologic features detected by OCT are being studied as possible prognostic indicators in ROP. Moreover, OCT might give us new measurable treatment assessment points.

Conflict of interest

The authors declare no conflict of interest.

Author details

Artemiy Kokhanov[1]*, Ye He[2], Pooja Nikki Bisarya[3] and Irena Tsui[2]

1 Paul L. Foster School of Medicine, Texas Tech University Health Sciences Center, El Paso, TX, USA

2 Stein Eye Institute and Doheny Eye Institute, University of California, Los Angeles, CA, USA

3 David Geffen School of Medicine, University of California, Los Angeles, CA, USA

*Address all correspondence to: akokhano@ttuhsc.edu

References

[1] Sommer A, Taylor HR, Ravilla TD, et al. Challenges of ophthalmic care in the developing world. JAMA Ophthalmology. 2014;**132**(5):640

[2] Terry TL. Extreme prematurity and fibroblastic overgrowth of persistent vascular sheath behind each crystalline lens. American Journal of Ophthalmology. 2018;**192**:xxviii

[3] Patz A, Hoeck LE, De La Cruz E. Studies on the effect of high oxygen administration in retrolental fibroplasia*. American Journal of Ophthalmology. 1952;**35**(9):1248-1253

[4] Parmelee AH, Pilger IS, Austin WO. Retrolental fibroplasia; a reduction in incidence following a decrease in use of oxygen therapy for premature infants. California Medicine. 1956;**84**(6):424-426

[5] Shah PK, Prabhu V, Karandikar SS, Ranjan R, Narendran V, Kalpana N. Retinopathy of prematurity: Past, present and future. World Journal of Clinical Pediatrics. 2016;**5**(1):35-46

[6] Vinekar A, Dogra M, Azad RV, Gilbert C, Gopal L, Trese M. The changing scenario of retinopathy of prematurity in middle and low income countries: Unique solutions for unique problems. Indian Journal of Ophthalmology. 2019;**67**(6):717-719

[7] Blencowe H, Lawn JE, Vazquez T, Fielder A, Gilbert C. Preterm-associated visual impairment and estimates of retinopathy of prematurity at regional and global levels for 2010. Pediatric Research. 2013;**74**(Suppl. 1):35-49

[8] Mangalesh S, McGeehan B, Tai V, et al. Macular oct characteristics at 36 weeks' postmenstrual age in infants examined for retinopathy of prematurity. Ophthalmology Retina. 2021;**5**(6):580-592

[9] Agarwal K, Vinekar A, Chandra P, et al. Imaging the pediatric retina: An overview. Indian Journal of Ophthalmology. 2021;**69**(4):812

[10] Patel CK. Optical coherence tomography in the management of acute retinopathy of prematurity. American Journal of Ophthalmology. 2006;**141**(3):582-584

[11] Joshi MM, Trese MT, Capone A. Optical coherence tomography findings in stage 4a retinopathy of prematurity. Ophthalmology. 2006;**113**(4):657-660

[12] Vinekar A, Avadhani K, Sivakumar M, et al. Understanding clinically undetected macular changes in early retinopathy of prematurity on spectral domain optical coherence tomography. Investigative Ophthalmology & Visual Science. 2011;**52**(8):5183

[13] Vinekar A, Sivakumar M, Shetty R, et al. A novel technique using spectral-domain optical coherence tomography (Spectralis, sd-oct+hra) to image supine non-anaesthetized infants: Utility demonstrated in aggressive posterior retinopathy of prematurity. Eye (London, England). 2010;**24**(2):379-382

[14] Kothari N, Chu A, Huang JM, et al. Arm-mounted optical coherence tomography angiography in extremely low birth weight neonates with retinopathy of prematurity. American Journal of Ophthalmology Case Reports. 2020;**18**:100624

[15] Maldonado RS, Izatt JA, Sarin N, et al. Optimizing hand-held spectral domain optical coherence tomography imaging for neonates, infants, and children. Investigative Ophthalmology & Visual Science. 2010;**51**(5):2678

[16] Cook A, White S, Batterbury M, Clark D. Ocular growth and refractive error development in premature infants with or without retinopathy of prematurity. Investigative Ophthalmology & Visual Science. 2008;**49**(12):5199-5207

[17] Maldonado RS, Toth CA. Optical coherence tomography in retinopathy of prematurity. Clinics in Perinatology. 2013;**40**(2):271-296

[18] Vural A, Perente İ, Onur İU, et al. Efficacy of intravitreal aflibercept monotherapy in retinopathy of prematurity evaluated by periodic fluorescence angiography and optical coherence tomography. International Ophthalmology. 2019;**39**(10):2161-2169

[19] Zhou K, Song S, Legocki A, et al. Quantitative handheld swept-source optical coherence tomography angiography in awake preterm and full-term infants. Translational Vision Science and Technology. 2020;**9**(13):19

[20] Moshiri Y, Legocki AT, Zhou K, et al. Handheld swept-source optical coherence tomography with angiography in awake premature neonates. Quantitative Imaging in Medicine and Surgery. 2019;**9**(9):1495502-1491502

[21] Nonobe N, Kaneko H, Ito Y, et al. Optical coherence tomography angiography of the foveal avascular zone in children with a history of treatment-requiring retinopathy of prematurity. Retina. 2019;**39**(1):111-117

[22] He Y, Pettenkofer M, Nittala MG, Sadda SR, Tsui I, Chu A. Early postnatal oxygen exposure predicts choroidal thinning in neonates. Investigative Ophthalmology & Visual Science. 2021;**62**(9):23

[23] Scruggs BA, Ni S, Nguyen TTP, et al. Peripheral oct assisted by scleral depression in retinopathy of prematurity. Ophthalmology Science. 2022;**2**(1):100094

[24] Mangalesh S, Sarin N, McGeehan B, et al. Preterm infant stress during handheld optical coherence tomography vs binocular indirect ophthalmoscopy examination for retinopathy of prematurity. JAMA Ophthalmology. 2021;**139**(5):567

[25] Nguyen TTP, Ni S, Ostmo S, et al. Association of optical coherence tomography–measured fibrovascular ridge thickness and clinical disease stage in retinopathy of prematurity. JAMA Ophthalmology. 2022;**140**(11):1121

[26] Nguyen TTP, Ni S, Khan S, et al. Advantages of widefield optical coherence tomography in the diagnosis of retinopathy of prematurity. Frontiers in Pediatrics. 2022;**9**:797684

[27] Chavala SH, Farsiu S, Maldonado R, Wallace DK, Freedman SF, Toth CA. Insights into advanced retinopathy of prematurity using handheld spectral domain optical coherence tomography imaging. Ophthalmology. 2009;**116**(12):2448-2456

[28] Wallace DK, Kylstra JA, Greenman DB, Freedman SF. Significance of isolated neovascular tufts ("popcorn") in retinopathy of prematurity. Journal of AAPOS. 1998;**2**(1):52-56

[29] Lee AC, Maldonado RS, Sarin N, et al. Macular features from spectral-domain optical coherence tomography as

an adjunct to indirect ophthalmoscopy in retinopathy of prematurity. Retina. 2011;**31**(8):1470-1482

[30] Zepeda EM, Shariff A, Gillette TB, et al. Vitreous bands identified by handheld spectral-domain optical coherence tomography among premature infants. JAMA Ophthalmology. 2018;**136**(7):753

[31] He Y, Chen X, Tsui I, Vajzovic L, Sadda SR. Insights into the developing fovea revealed by imaging. Progress in Retinal and Eye Research. 2022;**90**:101067

[32] Todorich B, Thanos A, Yonekawa Y, et al. Surgical management of tractional retinoschisis associated with vitreous hemorrhage in retinopathy of prematurity. Retinal Cases & Brief Reports. 2019;**13**(1):72-74

[33] O'Sullivan ML, Ying GS, Mangalesh S, et al. Foveal differentiation and inner retinal displacement are arrested in extremely premature infants. Investigative Ophthalmology & Visual Science. 2021;**62**(2):25

[34] He Y, Pettenkofer M, Chu A, Sadda SR, Corradetti G, Tsui I. Characterization of foveal development in treatment-naïve extremely preterm infants. Translational Vision Science & Technology. 2022;**11**(6):11

[35] Vajzovic L, Rothman AL, Tran-Viet D, Cabrera MT, Freedman SF, Toth CA. Delay in retinal photoreceptor development in very preterm compared to term infants. Investigative Ophthalmology & Visual Science. 2015;**56**(2):908-913

[36] Michalak SM, Mangalesh S, Shen LL, et al. Systemic factors associated with a thinner choroid in preterm infants. Ophthalmology Science. 2021;**1**(2):100032

[37] Moreno TA, O'Connell RV, Chiu SJ, et al. Choroid development and feasibility of choroidal imaging in the preterm and term infants utilizing SD-OCT. Investigative Ophthalmology & Visual Science. 2013;**54**(6):4140-4147

[38] Chen X, Prakalapakorn SG, Freedman SF, Vajzovic L, Toth CA. Differentiating retinal detachment and retinoschisis using handheld optical coherence tomography in stage 4 retinopathy of prematurity. JAMA Ophthalmology. 2020;**138**(1):81

[39] Lee H, Proudlock FA, Gottlob I. Pediatric optical coherence tomography in clinical practice—Recent progress. Investigative Ophthalmology & Visual Science. 2016;**57**(9):OCT69

[40] Cehajic-Kapetanovic J, Xue K, Purohit R, Patel CK. Flying baby optical coherence tomography alters the staging and management of advanced retinopathy of prematurity. Acta Ophthalmologica. 2021;**99**(4):441-447

[41] Muni RH, Kohly RP, Charonis AC, Lee TC. Retinoschisis detected with handheld spectral-domain optical coherence tomography in neonates with advanced retinopathy of prematurity. Archives of Ophthalmology. 2010;**128**(1):57-62

[42] Cabrera MT, Brewer EM, Grant L, Tarczy-Hornoch K. Exudative retinal detachment documented by handheld spectral domain optical coherence tomography after retinal laser photocoagulation for retinopathy of prematurity. Retinal Cases & Brief Reports. 2021;**15**(3):310-313

[43] The international classification of retinopathy of prematurity

revisited. Archives of Ophthalmology. 2005;**123**(7):991

[44] Seely KR, Wang KL, Tai V, et al. Auto-processed retinal vessel shadow view images from bedside optical coherence tomography to evaluate plus disease in retinopathy of prematurity. Translational Vision Science and Technology. 2020;**9**(9):16

[45] Maldonado RS, Yuan E, Tran-Viet D, et al. Three-dimensional assessment of vascular and perivascular characteristics in subjects with retinopathy of prematurity. Ophthalmology. 2014;**121**(6):1289-1296

[46] Dubis AM, Subramaniam CD, Godara P, Carroll J, Costakos DM. Subclinical macular findings in infants screened for retinopathy of prematurity with spectral-domain optical coherence tomography. Ophthalmology. 2013;**120**(8):1665-1671

[47] Maldonado RS, O'Connell R, Ascher SB, et al. Spectral-domain optical coherence tomographic assessment of severity of cystoid macular edema in retinopathy of prematurity. Archives of Ophthalmology. 2012;**130**(5):569-578

[48] Hee MR, Puliafito CA, Wong C, et al. Quantitative assessment of macular edema with optical coherence tomography. Archives of Ophthalmology. 1995;**113**(8):1019-1029

[49] Yanoff M, Fine BS, Brucker AJ, Eagle RC. Pathology of human cystoid macular edema. Survey of Ophthalmology. 1984;**28**(Suppl):505-511

[50] Sato T, Kusaka S, Shimojo H, Fujikado T. Simultaneous analyses of vitreous levels of 27 cytokines in eyes with retinopathy of prematurity. Ophthalmology. 2009;**116**(11):2165-2169

[51] Erol MK, Ozdemir O, Turgut Coban D, et al. Macular findings obtained by spectral domain optical coherence tomography in retinopathy of prematurity. Journal of Ophthalmology. 2014;**2014**:1-7

[52] Jabroun MN, AlWattar BK, Fulton AB. Optical coherence tomography angiography in prematurity. Seminars in Ophthalmology. 2021;**36**(4):264-269

[53] Anwar S, Nath M, Patel A, et al. Potential utility of foveal morphology in preterm infants measured using hand-held optical coherence tomography in retinopathy of prematurity screening. Retina. 2020;**40**(8):1592-1602

[54] Rothman AL, Tran-Viet D, Gustafson KE, et al. Poorer neurodevelopmental outcomes associated with cystoid macular edema identified in preterm infants in the intensive care nursery. Ophthalmology. 2015;**122**(3):610-619

[55] Vinekar A, Mangalesh S, Jayadev C, Maldonado RS, Bauer N, Toth CA. Retinal imaging of infants on spectral domain optical coherence tomography. BioMed Research International. 2015;**2015**:e782420

[56] Tong AY, El-Dairi M, Maldonado RS, et al. Evaluation of optic nerve development in preterm and term infants using handheld spectral-domain optical coherence tomography. Ophthalmology. 2014;**121**(9):1818-1826

[57] Mataftsi A, Dermenoudi M, Dastiridou A, et al. Optical coherence tomography angiography in children with spontaneously regressed retinopathy of prematurity. Eye. 2021;**35**(5):1411-1417

[58] Bowl W, Stieger K, Bokun M, et al. Oct-based macular structure-function

correlation in dependence on birth weight and gestational age-the giessen long-term rop study. Investigative Ophthalmology & Visual Science. 2016;**57**(9):OCT235-OCT241

[59] Tariq YM, Burlutsky G, Mitchell P. Macular parameters and prematurity: A spectral domain coherence tomography study. Journal of American Association for Pediatric Ophthalmology and Strabismus. 2012;**16**(4):382-385

[60] Lenis TL, Gunzenhauser RC, Fung SSM, et al. Myopia and anterior segment optical coherence tomography findings in laser-treated retinopathy of prematurity eyes. Journal of American Association for Pediatric Ophthalmology and Strabismus. 2020;**24**(2):86.e1-86.e7

[61] Morken TS, Dammann O, Skranes J, Austeng D. Retinopathy of prematurity, visual and neurodevelopmental outcome, and imaging of the central nervous system. Seminars in Perinatology. 2019;**43**(6):381-389

[62] Czeszyk A, Hautz W, Jaworski M, Bulsiewicz D, Czech-Kowalska J. Morphology and vessel density of the macula in preterm children using optical coherence tomography angiography. Journal of Clinical Medicine. 2022;**11**(5):1337

[63] Falavarjani KG, Iafe NA, Velez FG, et al. Optical coherence tomography angiography of the fovea in children born preterm. Retina. 2017;**37**(12):2289-2294

[64] Balasubramanian S, Borrelli E, Lonngi M, et al. Visual function and optical coherence tomography angiography features in children born preterm. Retina. 2019;**39**(11):2233-2239

[65] Chen YC, Chen YT, Chen SN. Foveal microvascular anomalies on optical coherence tomography angiography and the correlation with foveal thickness and visual acuity in retinopathy of prematurity. Graefe's Archive for Clinical and Experimental Ophthalmology. 2019;**257**(1):23-30

[66] Periti F, Toma C, Plaitano C, et al. Microvascular parameters evaluated with optical coherence tomography-angiography in children: Comparison between preterm and full-term patients. Acta Ophthalmologica. 2019;**97**(7):e1032-e1034

[67] Rezar-Dreindl S, Eibenberger K, Told R, et al. Retinal vessel architecture in retinopathy of prematurity and healthy controls using swept-source optical coherence tomography angiography. Acta Ophthalmologica. 2021;**99**(2):e232-e239

[68] Park KA, Oh SY. Analysis of spectral-domain optical coherence tomography in preterm children: Retinal layer thickness and choroidal thickness profiles. Investigative Ophthalmology & Visual Science. 2012;**53**(11):7201

[69] Villegas VM. Widefield optical coherence tomography of foveal dragging in retinopathy of prematurity. International Journal of Ophthalmology. 2019;**12**(7):1219-1223

Section 2

Optical Coherence Tomography and Optic Nerve

Chapter 5

The Role of Optical Coherence Tomography Angiography in Glaucoma

Karanjit Kooner, Mahad Rehman, Sruthi Suresh, Emily Buchanan, Mohannad Albdour and Hafsa Zuberi

Abstract

Glaucoma is the second leading cause of blindness worldwide, affecting eighty million people globally and three million patients in the USA. Primary open-angle glaucoma, the most common type, is a multifactorial progressive optic nerve neurodegenerative disorder that leads to loss of optic nerve head (ONH) tissue, thinning of the retinal nerve fiber layer, and corresponding visual field (VF) defects with or without elevated intraocular pressure (IOP). Risk factors include older age, black or Hispanic race, elevated IOP, thin central corneal thickness, disk hemorrhage, and low ocular perfusion pressure. The two prevalent theories explaining glaucomatous damage are mechanical (elevated IOP) and vascular (compromised optic nerve perfusion). Current diagnostic methods, such as measuring IOP, VF testing, and ONH evaluation, are subjective and often unreliable. Optical coherence tomography angiography (OCTA) is a rapid, non-invasive imaging modality that provides 3-D, volumetric details of both the structure and vascular networks of the retina and optic nerve. Various researchers have shown that OCTA provides an accurate and objective evaluation of the retina and the optic nerve in glaucoma. This chapter describes the role of OCTA in managing patients with glaucoma.

Keywords: optical coherence tomography angiography, glaucoma, intraocular pressure, optic nerve, visual field

1. Introduction

1.1 Overview of glaucoma

Glaucoma is the second leading cause of blindness which affects over 80 million people worldwide [1]. Of the various subtypes of glaucoma, the most common is primary open-angle glaucoma (POAG), a multifactorial, progressive optic neuropathy characterized by cupping of the optic nerve head (ONH) and visual field (VF) defects with or without elevated intraocular pressure (IOP) [2]. Glaucomatous optic neuropathy is driven pathologically by degeneration of the retinal ganglion cells (RGCs) and atrophy of the retinal nerve fiber layer (RNFL) (**Figure 1**).

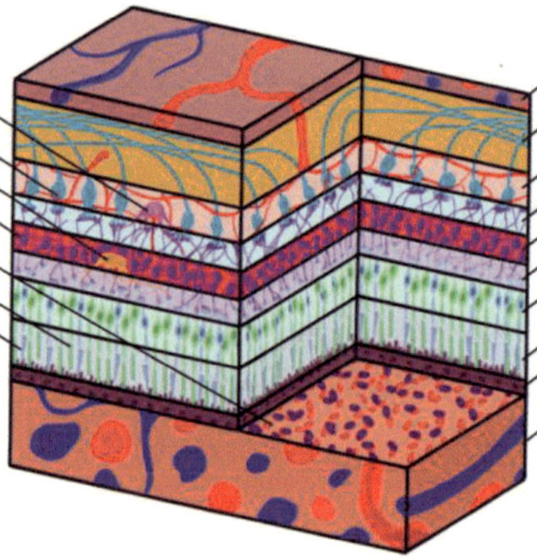

Figure 1.
Cross-section of the retina illustrating the retinal layers and underlying vascular supply in a healthy eye.

Early work in 1858 by German anatomist Heinrich Mueller led to the concept of the mechanical theory: elevated IOP leads to the compression of optic nerve fibers at the level of the lamina cribrosa which in turn causes blockages to the axoplasmic flow [3]. In the same year, another German scientist, Eduard von Jaeger proposed an alternative vascular theory where he suggested that the underlying cause of optic nerve damage was due to poor perfusion to the ONH with or without elevated IOP [4]. Today, it is widely accepted that glaucoma being a multifactorial disease may be consistent with both the mechanical and vascular models. Schematics in **Figures 2** and **3** show the pathological changes a human eye undergoes during glaucoma as per the vascular and mechanical theories.

1.2 Optical coherence tomography angiography addresses current challenges in glaucoma diagnosis

Glaucoma is diagnosed using three parameters: measurement of IOP, evaluation of the optic nerve anatomy, and VF testing. However, this approach is limited by its inherent subjectivity and measurement inconsistencies. One key challenge is that IOP measurement is not standardized and can be affected by the central corneal thickness (CCT), type of tonometer used, time of day, as well as the skill and training of the clinical staff obtaining the measurements. Similarly, visual assessment of the optic nerve and VF testing are subject to high degrees of inter- and intra-examiner variation, limiting their abilities to diagnose and follow patients with glaucoma accurately and objectively.

Due to these challenges, optical coherence tomography (OCT) technology has grown in popularity due to its ability to provide additional objective information about the structure and morphology of the optic nerve and retina. Specifically, peripapillary retinal nerve fiber layer (RNFL) analysis is widely used for glaucoma diagnosis, as RNFL thinning can indicate glaucomatous damage [5]. While OCT has greatly improved the accuracy and consistency of glaucoma diagnosis, it is still limited since it cannot probe the vascular degradation that occurs in glaucoma. Particularly, it is extremely challenging to distinguish between differing degrees of glaucoma severity, identify patients with optic cupping who have normal vascular perfusion, as well as monitor patient response to treatment over time.

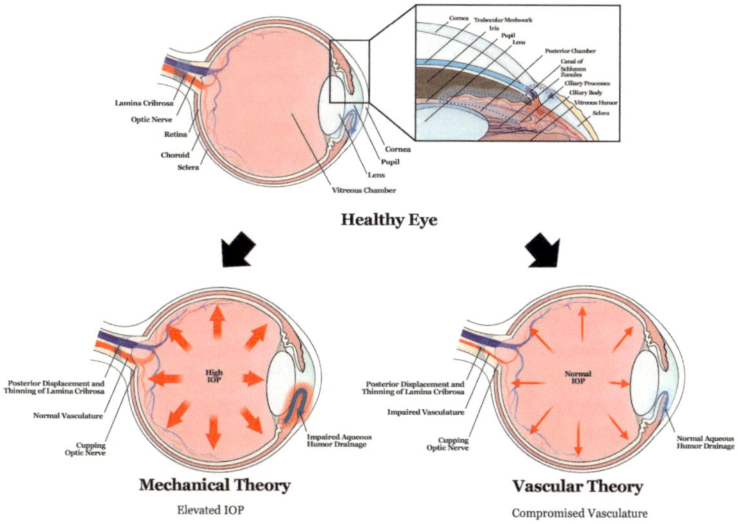

Figure 2.
Aqueous humor dynamics in the healthy (top) and glaucomatous (bottom) eye as hypothesized by the mechanical theory (left) and vascular theory (right).

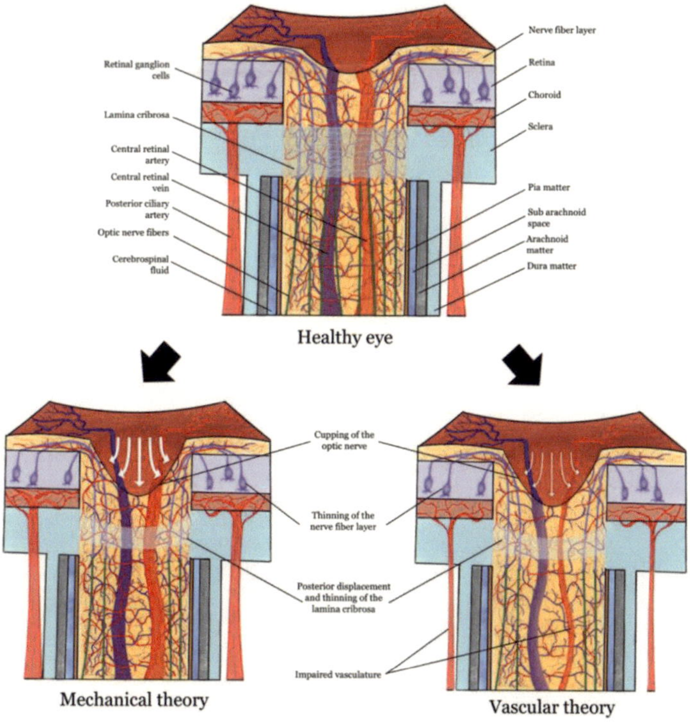

Figure 3.
Cross section of the optic nerve in the healthy (top) and the glaucomatous (bottom) eye as hypothesized by the mechanical theory (left) and vascular theory (right).

Improvements in the OCT technology has led to the development of optical coherence tomography angiography (OCTA), a rapid, noninvasive imaging modality that can provide quantitative and volumetric assessment of both the structure and vascular aspects of the retinal and optic nerve. Thus, OCTA has addressed prior limitations of OCT and has revolutionized the evaluation of several ophthalmic diseases, including glaucoma by allowing clinicians to distinguish between glaucoma suspect, healthy, and glaucomatous eyes [6–9].

2. Optical coherence tomography angiography

2.1 The development of optical coherence tomography

OCT technology was first developed at the Massachusetts Institute of Technology by David Huang in 1991 [10] (**Figure 4**). It is a non-invasive imaging methodology for acquiring high resolution images of the retina and optic nerve using low-coherence interferometry. In this technique a beam of light is shone into the eye and reflected light is captured and measured. By comparing the reflected light to an unobstructed reference path, the location and morphology of ocular structures can be determined to generate a cross sectional image of the eye [10, 25]. This imaging modality provides key structural information such as retinal thickness (µm), RNFL thickness (µm), and abnormal reflectivity on retinal layers which could indicate the presence of edema, exudates, calcifications, or atrophy [26, 27]. Thus, OCT technology introduced a novel and precise method for visualizing and measuring defects in the optic nerve, retina, and nerve fiber layer. Soon after the publication of the first images of the optic disk, Humphrey instruments introduced the first commercial OCT scanner in 1996 [11]. Ten years later, Optovue's spectral domain (SD-OCT) scanner was the first to obtain FDA approval for clinical use [12].

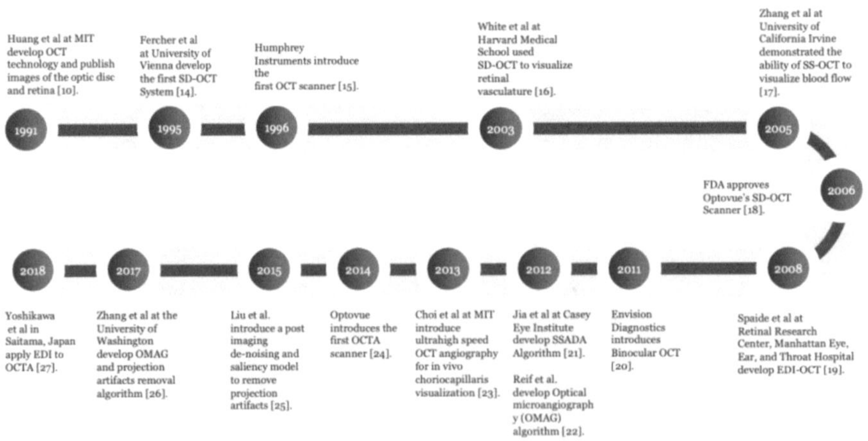

Figure 4.
Milestones in the development of optical coherence tomography angiography [10–24].

2.2 The development of optical coherence tomography angiography

Although OCT can provide information about the structure of the retina and the optic nerve, it is unable to assess the vascular impairment and degradation known to play a key role in glaucoma pathophysiology. To fully assess damage in glaucoma patients, additional details about the retina and optic nerve vasculature are needed.

Initial work by White et al. showed that SD- OCT could be used to probe the retinal vasculature and was expanded upon by Zhang et al. who used a technique called swept source (SS) OCT to visualize blood flow in 2005 [14, 15]. This was accomplished by repeatedly scanning a transverse cross-sectional area of the retina and analyzing the scan differences caused by movement [6]. Since the presence of blood flow creates movement which affects the reflectance in each scan, successive scans or "angiograms" can be used to probe the underlying vasculature of the eye.

In 2018, Nesper et al. demonstrated the complexity and connectivity of parafoveal capillary plexuses and identified the location of specific arterioles seen in prior histological studies [28]. This enhanced understanding of vasculature and their perfusion greatly improved the assessment of many ophthalmological diseases, including glaucoma.

Work in the past decade has focused on accurately delineating blood vessels by employing sophisticated algorithms. In 2012 Reif et al. introduced a phase-based algorithm known as optical microangiography (OMAG), which uses intensity and phase information from repeated B-scans to delineate blood vessels [19]. In the same year, Spaide et al. showed that an amplitude-based method called split-spectrum amplitude decorrelation angiography (SSADA) could delineate blood vessels by measuring the decorrelation between two consecutive B-scans [6]. Research has found SSADA to be superior in the detection and connectivity of microvascular networks compared to other algorithms [18]. Current investigations of OCTA technology aim to implement novel deep learning (DL) and machine learning (ML) techniques to reduce or remove image artifacts to enhance OCTA accuracy.

3. Optical coherence tomography angiography in glaucoma

3.1 Optical coherence tomography angiography metrics for glaucoma evaluation

Early OCTA work in glaucoma by Jia et al. in 2012, was limited to the observation and quantification of the optic disk alone (disk flow index and disk perfusion) [29]. As this technology has progressed, a broad range of OCTA metrics were introduced to quantify microvasculature and aid in the diagnosis of glaucoma. Specifically, density parameters are used to track disease progression [18, 30–33] and more recent work has explored how changes in the macular regions, foveal avascular zone (FAZ), and deep retinal layer microvasculature contribute to disease severity [9].

Current clinical evaluations of glaucoma using OCTA rely predominantly on eight parameters: RNFL (μm), cup/disk ratio (CDR), macular ganglion cell complex (mGCC) in μm, focal loss volume (FLV, %), global loss volume (GLV, %), whole image ONH vessel density (VD, %), whole image macular VD, (%), and FAZ area (mm^2). Recently, a key study by AlSalem et al. explored the efficacy of each of these metrics for classifying the severity of glaucoma progression into three categories: mild, moderate, severe [9]. Their parameter classifications are summarized in **Table 1**. Of note, the authors described how severe cases of POAG showed a

Variables	Controls (n = 69) (%)	Mild Glaucoma (n = 54) (%)	Moderate Glaucoma (n = 25) (%)	Severe Glaucoma (n = 12) (%)	P value* (All groups)
RNFL (µm)	96.11 ± 9.80	82.95 ± 11.75	76.91 ± 14.45	60.13 ± 7.51	<0.01
CDR	0.49 ± 0.14	0.54 ± 0.15	0.57 ± 0.17	0.73 ± 0.12	<0.01
mGCC Average (µm)	94.29 ± 9.65	83.71 ± 8.65	80.31 ± 14.99	67.92 ± 10.90	<0.01
FLV (%)	1.08 ± 1.21	2.93 ± 3.46	6.12 ± 3.92	9.39 ± 4.03	<0.01
GLV (%)	4.53 ± 4.78	12.37 ± 7.82	17.05 ± 11.31	29.39 ± 8.89	<0.01
Whole Image ONH Vessel Density (%)	56.71 ± 4.36	52.85 ± 5.15	49.82 ± 4.06	43.12 ± 4.19	<0.01
Whole Image Macular Vessel Density (%)	50.27 ± 4.23	48.12 ± 3.80	46.13 ± 3.91	43.43 ± 4.71	<0.01
FAZ Area (mm^2)	0.34 ± 0.14	0.33 ± 0.14	0.40 ± 0.16	0.36 ± 0.16	0.51

Table 1.
Structural and vessel density characteristics of healthy controls and glaucomatous eyes, adapted from AlSalem et al. [9].

significant decrease in signal strength intensity (SSI) for RNFL and ONH VD scans, whereas four parameters (whole image ONH VD, whole image macular VD, average RNFL thickness, and average mGCC thickness) decreased in a stepwise fashion as glaucoma progressed. These findings enable researchers to use both structural and VD parameters as indicators of glaucoma severity, adding new prognostic metrics that could not be obtained through VF tests alone.

3.1.1 Optical coherence tomography angiography features of the optic nerve head in glaucoma

Evaluation of the ONH microcirculation is commonly used to detect vascular damage in the glaucomatous eye, as there is a significant correlation between glaucoma severity and degree of VD loss in this region [9]. While the ONH of a healthy eye displays a dense microvascular network with no focal capillary dropout and a full RNFL thickness, the ONH microcirculation of a glaucomatous eye shows decreased perfusion and loss of the RNFL [9, 18].

In 2012, Jia et al. developed the SSADA algorithm to visualize and quantify ONH microcirculation [18]. In this pilot study, the SSADA results were applied to patients with early glaucoma to detect ONH perfusion abnormalities. The researchers found that ONH flow index and VD in patients with early glaucoma were significantly reduced compared to healthy controls. Furthermore, the ONH perfusion defects preceded VF changes, aiding in the early detection of disease.

Four years later, Chen et al. used OMAG-based OCTA to evaluate ONH blood vessels and perfusion and found that ONH perfusion decline was significantly correlated to the presence of structural and functional defects as well as disease severity [30]. Recently, Eslami et al. showed that OCTA ONH parameters can also discriminate between stages of glaucoma. Their cross-sectional investigation of patients with moderate and advanced glaucoma found that the VD of the inferior hemifield of the ONH area had the best performance in discriminating POAG stages [33].

3.2 Optical coherence tomography angiography features of the peripapillary region in glaucoma

Compared to healthy eyes, glaucomatous eyes show significantly lower peripapillary VD and blood flow index. A systematic review conducted by Bekkers et al. determined that the peripapillary microvasculature zone was the most discriminative region to aid glaucoma diagnosis as it provided an area under receiver operator characteristic curve AUROC of 0.8. [32]. Further gains in AUROC were obtained when model parameters were constricted to the superficial capillary plexus within the peripapillary region (AUROC =0.87).

Later work by De Jesus et al. confirmed that the superficial layer of the peripapillary region was the most useful OCTA metric to discern a glaucoma diagnosis, as damage was most prominent in this zone of the eye when compared to healthy controls [31]. Thus, analyzing the peripapillary region is a powerful application of OCTA as it provides the highest discriminant power to differentiate between healthy and glaucomatous eyes.

3.3 Optical coherence tomography angiography features of the macula in glaucoma

The macula is an area of great interest in glaucoma since it contains the highest density of RGCs. These multilayered cells are believed to be damaged early in the disease process [34]. Not only does a correlation exist between mean macular thickness and VF sensitivity, but the macular region has also been shown to have a significantly lower VD and blood flow index in patients with glaucoma compared to healthy controls [31].

In an age-matched study, Takusagawa et al. assessed macular thickness and circulation in patients with preperimetric glaucoma (PPG) and found that they had significant macular perfusion defects compared to healthy controls [35]. The authors additionally found that within the macular region, the hemispheric superficial vascular complex (SVC) VD values were highly correlated with the corresponding GCC thickness and VF sensitivity in glaucoma patients. Their landmark findings indicate that early in the disease process, glaucoma preferentially affects perfusion in the SVC of the macula rather than the deeper plexuses.

3.4 Optical coherence tomography angiography features of the choroidal microvasculature in glaucoma

According to vascular theory, changes in the choroidal microvasculature may play a key role in the pathophysiology of glaucoma as it supplies nutrition to both the optic nerve and the outer layers of retina. In a study evaluating parapapillary choroidal microvasculature dropout (MVD), Kim et al. found that MVD was associated with progressive RNFL thinning and worsening VF parameters [36]. The authors proposed that progressive retinal ganglion cell damage decreases metabolic demand and leads to reduced vascular perfusion and more extensive MVD.

Recently, Chatziralli et al. found that the peripapillary and MVD were lower in eyes with pseudoexfoliative glaucoma (PXG) [37]. This indicates optic nerve hypoperfusion may play a greater role in patients with PXG.

3.5 Using optical coherence tomography angiography to monitor disease progression in glaucoma

OCTA may have a role in the early detection and monitoring of the progression of glaucoma progression. AlSalem et al. found that whole image ONH VD, whole image macular VD, average RNFL thickness, average mGCC thickness, and cataract status were predictive of worsening VF MD [9]. They also determined that structural properties and VD were equally effective at determining the glaucomatous stage. This was supported by the findings of Geyman et al. and Chen et al. who also determined that structural properties and VD values were equally effective at determining the glaucoma stage [38, 39]. Tracking the previously described OCTA parameters over time may enable physicians to objectively gauge glaucoma progression.

3.6 Use of optical coherence tomography angiography in healthy, glaucoma suspect, and eyes with POAG

Using a standard OCTA protocol, typical qualitative and quantitative findings in healthy, glaucoma suspects, and eyes with POAG are shown in **Figure 5**. A, E, and I are images of the ONH and corresponding CDR. The B, F, and J show a map of the superficial retinal vessels and VD in different zones around the macula. C, G, and K show the nerve fiber layer thickness in the corresponding zones. D, H, and L are area maps of the radial peripapillary capillary VD.

The healthy eye (5A-D) has normal retinal morphology and OCTA parameter values. The CDR is 0.35, the retinal VD is 46%, the RNFL thickness is 113 μm, and the peripapillary capillary density is 53%. In a glaucoma suspect eye (5E-H), the enlarged CDR (0.80) alone may mislead the clinician. However, OCTA measurements of the VD (43%), RNFL (115 μm), and peripapillary capillary density (54%) are in the normal range. The OCTA scans of an eye with POAG (5I-L) show several abnormal findings characteristic of glaucoma. There is a severe degree of cupping (CDR 0.85), the overall retinal VD is reduced to 34%, the RNFL thickness is 55 μm, and the radial peripapillary VD is 34%.

3.7 Using optical coherence tomography angiography to characterize myopia

In clinical practice, detecting glaucoma in myopic patients has always been extremely challenging. As myopia increases, findings such as ONH tilt, increased ovality of the ONH, and peripapillary atrophy become more prominent [40]. The peripapillary RNFL thickness peaks also shift in myopic eyes, leading to difficulties in detecting thinning (40. Examples of changes seen in a patient with moderate myopia are shown in **Figure 6**.

In patients with high myopia, OCTA can be helpful in identifying the narrowing of vessel diameters which leads to reduced retinal VD and indirectly implying impaired blood flow. Suwan et al. found that patients with myopia alone had lower peripapillary VD compared to healthy controls [41]. Furthermore, patients with both myopia and glaucoma had an even greater reduction in VD that allowed the researchers to distinguish these patients from healthy controls, myopia only patients, and patients with glaucoma alone [41].

Recent work by Chang et al. found that both peripapillary and macular perfusion density were significantly reduced in patients with high myopia (HM) compared to non-high myopic (NHM) healthy controls [42]. However, macular perfusion

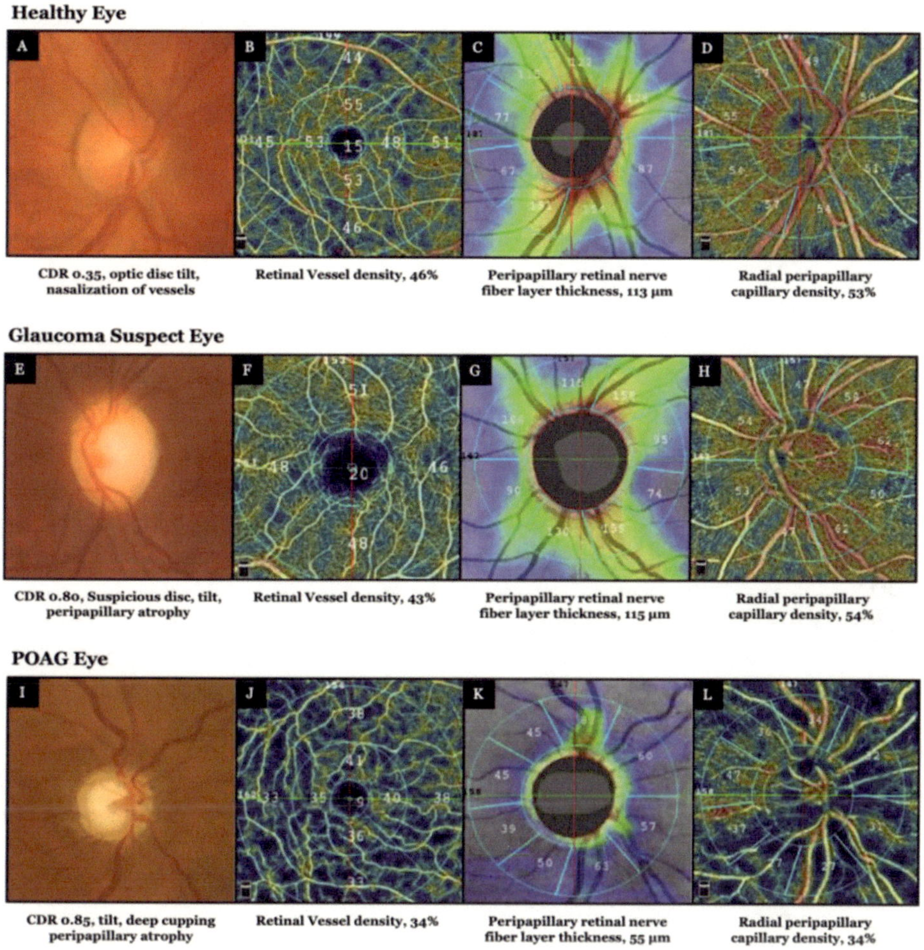

Figure 5.
Comparison of OCTA scans in healthy, glaucoma suspect, and eyes with POAG captured using the RTVue XR Avanti scanner (SSADA algorithm).

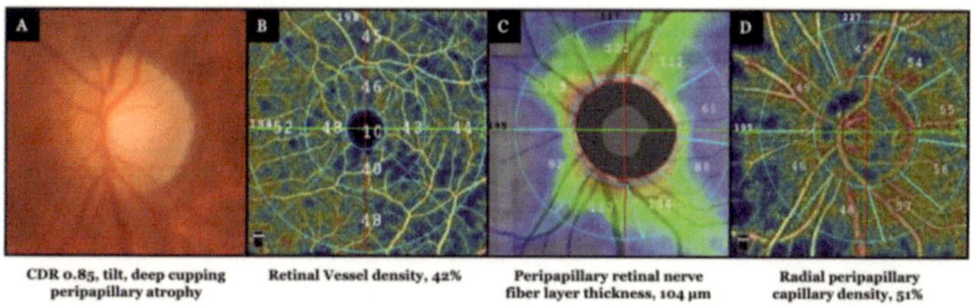

Figure 6.
OCTA scans from a non-glaucomatous myopic eye captured using the RTVue XR Avanti scanner (SSADA algorithm).

density was not decreased between patients with and without HM and could not be used for accurate diagnosis. They recommended that both macular OCTA and OCT imaging may be useful in diagnosing early glaucoma in patients with myopia. Shin et al. showed that peripapillary VD correlated more with VF mean sensitivity than peripapillary RNFL thickness and peripapillary perfusion density was significantly lower in patients with high myopia [43].

Bowd et al. took a different approach and created a novel *en face* texture-based analysis method to accurately discriminate between highly myopic glaucomatous and healthy eyes using macular tissue thickness measurements [40]. Their success was most likely due to the minimal tissue segmentation required in their approach compared to prior multilayer segmentation methods that often fail in highly myopic eyes. Another method by Yilmaz et al. found that utilizing a myopic normative database for peripapillary RNFL was very helpful in assessing differences in patients with varying degrees of myopia or when glaucoma co-existed with myopia [44]. Altogether, these recent works indicate that OCTA technology may improve the accuracy of glaucoma detection in patients with high myopia.

4. Limitations of optical coherence tomography angiography

Image artifacts are frequently encountered in OCTA and can hinder the interpretability of the microvascular structure and VD. In addition, media opacities and pupillary size can similarly affect the quality of OCTA maps and the calculation of VDs. Optimizing interscan time can also present a challenge in OCTA. While short capture times cannot detect slow flow velocities such as those observed in cases of venous occlusions [45], long interscan times are more sensitive to motion artifacts. Lastly, the lack of standardization across different devices and protocols remains a lingering limitation. For example, different commercially available OCTA devices differ in their methods of segmentation of the angiography slabs and axial and lateral resolutions [46].

4.1 Image artifacts in optical coherence tomography angiography

Image artifacts may be the result of errors during image acquisition, processing, and analysis and may be either patient related (**Figure** 7) or machine/operator related (**Figure 8**) [46].

4.1.1 Patient-related motion artifacts

One common cause of image artifacts is from eye movements caused by breathing, palpitations, or tremors (**Figure** 7). In general, eye movement artifacts appear as thin horizontal or vertical white lines (7A). They may cause duplication or removal of the retinal vessels shown in the image leading to an overall loss of vessel integrity. Blink

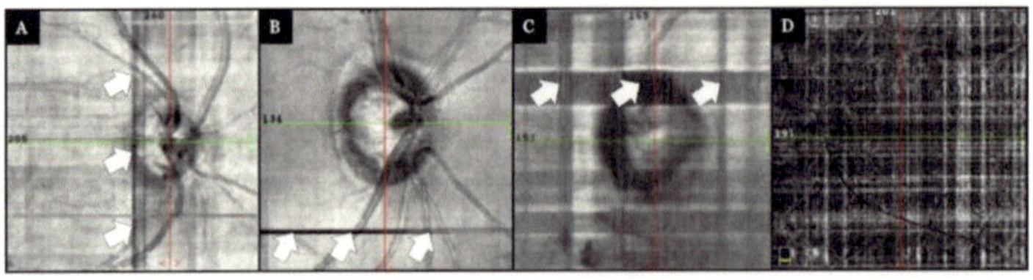

Figure 7.
Examples of patient related motion artifacts.

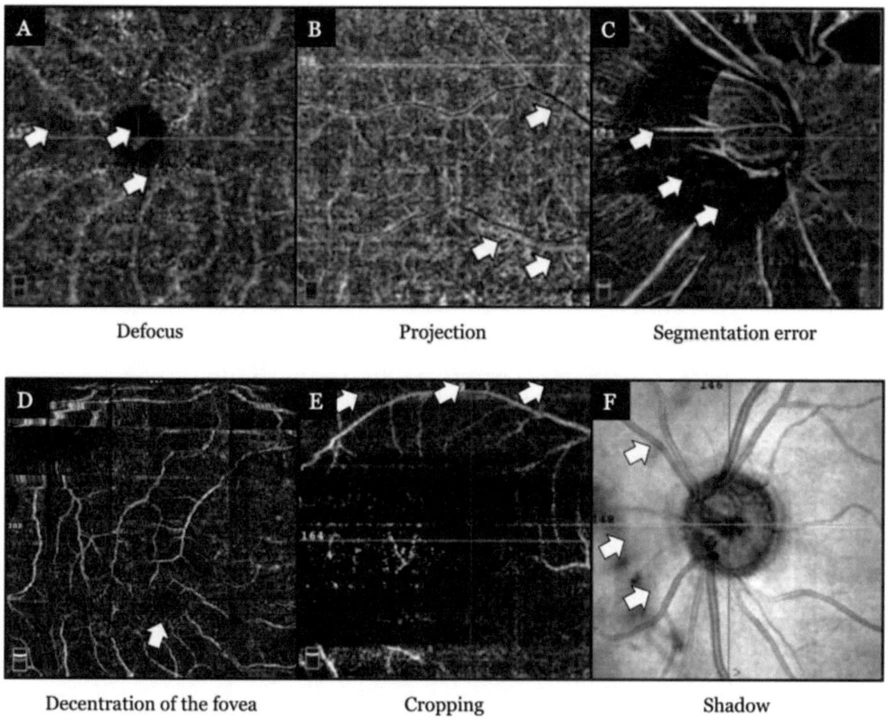

Figure 8.
Examples of operator or motion related OCTA artifacts.

artifacts occur when a patient blinks during scan capture which causes loss of reflectance intensity in an area of adjacent B-scans (7B). The displacement of multiple B-scans can cause horizontal or vertical black lines on the *en-face* angiogram. Refraction error, also described as banding, is caused by a temporary change in corneal refractive power when the patient-device distance fluctuates during acquisition (7 C). Criss-cross is an eye movement artifact that appears as a rectangular pattern when the software fails to correct multiple saccades (7D).

4.1.2 Operator/machine-related motion artifacts

There are several operator/machine related artifacts that affect the accuracy and precision of OCTA measurements. Poorly focused images cause defocused artifacts (8A) that are caused by a decrease in reflective intensity resulting in reduced definition of retinal microvasculature Projection artifacts (8B) occur when the shadow of vessels in the superficial layer imprint onto the deeper layer. Segmentation errors (8C) are produced when the automated segmentation algorithm inaccurately identifies the layers of the retina or optic nerve. Decentration artifact (8D) occurs if the fovea or ONH is translocated to the periphery of the scan, preventing the algorithm from correctly identifying these areas. Cropping (8E) refers to loss in image data caused by B-scan not being fully within the capture window. Lastly, vitreous floaters may result in shadow artifacts (8F) because of decreased intensity of retinal layers in focused areas and may prevent clear visualization of structures in the affected area.

4.1.3 Key factors that produce optical coherence tomography angiography artifacts

Since OCTA artifacts may affect the accuracy of glaucoma diagnosis it is important to understand when and why these alterations are likely to occur. Older patients often have poor-quality scans due to a higher frequency of media opacities such as cataracts and age-related retinal pathologies. Recently Kamalipour et al. showed that 40% of OCTA images in the glaucoma group had poorer quality compared to healthy controls [47]. This was confirmed by Cheng et al. who found that the presence of glaucoma significantly increased the odds for the presence of any artifacts [48]. Similarly, patients with glaucoma were found to have two times the odds of incorrect automatic segmentation of the retinal superficial layer even after adjustment for age and VF loss [48]. Image quality was also found to decrease as glaucoma progressed. Declining retinal thickness reduces the signal intensity of reflected waves causing increased prevalence of artifacts.

4.1.4 Prevalence of optical coherence tomography angiography artifacts

In a well-diversified population of North Texas consisting of 292 patients, Mekala et al. found that most patients (99.3%) had at least one artifact [49]. The most common artifacts were due to eye movements (66.1%), defocus (64.7%) and shadows (40%). The most severe (affecting more than 10% of the scan area) were seen in patients with POAG (31.4%) and myopia (30.75%). A similar study by Weijing et al. found that 88.34% of images had at least one artifact, the most common of which was projection (100%), followed by motion (75.22%), blur (24.78%) and decentration (21.28%) [50]. Another study by Kamalipour et al. excluded 33.9% of scans due to poor image quality and found that 13.6% had one artifact and 9.8% had two or more. In this study the most common artifact was eye movement (10.6%), followed by defocus (9.6%), correctable segmentation errors (7.6%), and uncorrectable segmentation errors (5.4%) [48]. Given that multiple studies have confirmed the presence of artifacts in a significant percentage of images, it is crucial to account for artifacts when evaluating OCTA in a clinical setting.

4.1.5 Current methods for reducing optical coherence tomography angiography artifacts

Eye tracking technology was first introduced in 2004 as a way to compensate for eye movement and improve the quality of OCT scans [51]. Since then, this technology has shown to decrease the odds of acquiring poor-quality images by half [47]. It is highly effective in reducing eye movement and defocus artifacts but does not currently decrease the occurrence of segmentation artifacts.

Work by Venugopal et al. found that high-density (HD) scans, which increase sampling density from 304 × 304 A-scans to 400 × 400 A-scans, showed significantly greater VD values and fewer poor-quality scans than non-HD scans [52]. Thus, both eye tracking technology and HD scanning are proven methods for reducing the presence of OCTA artifacts. However, additional work is needed to further reduce the prevalence of other artifacts in OCTA.

4.2 Repeatability and reproducibility challenges in optical coherence tomography angiography

OCTA's use is slowly becoming popular among clinicians for the diagnosis and monitoring of glaucoma. There are a number of commercially available OCTA devices including RTVue XR Avanti (Visionix USA Inc., previously Optovue Inc., Lombard, IL), Cirrus 5000 (Carl Zeiss Meditec Inc., Dublin, CA), PLEX Elite 9000 (Carl Zeiss Meditec Inc., Dublin, CA), and SPECTRALIS 2 (Heidelberg Engineering, Heidelberg, Germany). These devices all vary in terms of scan speed, wavelengths, eye tracking, image size, and vessel delineation algorithms. Differences in scan parameters and methodologies have led to discrepancies between images that limit direct comparisons across multiple centers and studies.

Several investigators have evaluated intra and inter-visit repeatability and of OCTA measurements in the ONH, peripapillary, and macular regions. Manalastas et al. compared the reproducibility of VD measurements between healthy and glaucoma eyes using the coefficient of variation (CV) the relative dispersion of data points around the mean, with a lower number indicating less variation [53]. The authors found that the CV of intra- and inter-visit global VD measures in healthy eyes ranged from 2.5–9.0% in macular scans and 1.8–3.2% in ONH scans, while the CV was higher in glaucoma (3.2–7.9% in macular scans vs. 2.3–4.1% in ONH scans. Venugopal et al. described similar results for peripapillary region (normal 2.5–4.4% vs. glaucoma 2.6–6.6%) and macular region (normal 3.3–4.7% vs. glaucoma 3.7–5.6%) [51]. Together, these studies suggest that glaucoma patients have sparser VD with slightly poorer reproducibility than healthy subjects [52].

Manalastas et al. examined the intra-visit and inter-visit reproducibility of SD-OCT RNFL thickness and GCC thickness in the scans from the prior studies [53]. The CVs of the global RNFL and GCC thickness were ≤ 4%, and the superior and inferior RNFL and GCC ≤ 3.5% in both healthy and glaucoma eyes. In agreement with the prior VD studies, glaucomatous eyes had worse RNFL and GCC reproducibility than healthy eyes ($p < 0.001$). The reproducibility of the global VD measures provided by OCTA is slightly worse than that of RNFL and GCC measures traditionally found in OCT.

AlSalem et al. studied reproducibility between patients across all stages of POAG and concluded that the range of CV for structural properties was greater than VD as glaucoma progressed [9]. Thus, as VD provides better reproducibility than structural values it may be a more consistent metric in severe POAG.

5. The future of optical coherence tomography angiography in glaucoma

Recently, artificial intelligence (AI) techniques such as machine learning (ML) and deep learning (DL) are increasingly being used in conjunction with OCTA to improve glaucoma diagnosis and track disease progression. However, further work is required to standardize the nomenclature and datasets utilized for ML and DL to maximize the impact of AI technology in OCTA.

5.1 Standardization of optical coherence tomography angiography

A major barrier that has prevented the compilation of large OCTA databases for ML and DL is the lack of standardization among OCTA instruments, imaging protocols, data analysis methods, and inconsistent nomenclature. This has made it very challenging to apply new technologies or methods to analyze data from different OCTA scanners and ophthalmology clinics. Therefore, establishing standardized protocols for imaging, data analysis, and terminology is crucial [54, 55].

5.2 Machine learning using optical coherence tomography angiography imaging

5.2.1 Overview of machine learning methodology

Broadly speaking, AI refers to computer science techniques which simulate human cognitive processes such as visual perception, speech recognition, and decision-making. ML is a subfield of AI that allows software systems to automatically learn and improve from experience without being explicitly programmed through the use of algorithms and statistical models that analyze and draw inferences from patterns in data. It involves training a model on a dataset and allowing the model to make predictions or decisions without human intervention [56, 57].

ML requires four sequential steps: an input of high-volume and high-quality data, extraction of features, model building, and performance evaluation [56]. The quality of the manual feature extraction from a dataset to be used as an input for ML is critical for optimal model performance. During this process, unique properties and patterns are identified which the model then uses to learn how to perform the task. These can include higher level features, such as glaucomatous eyes, or lower-level features such as image edges and shapes. The main caveat to high quality feature extraction is that it requires large data sets and many hours of precise identification of objects of interest by the researchers. One approach to reduce this burden is to use DL automated feature learning, where the model learns to extract and identify relevant features from a dataset automatically, without human intervention.

Once the features have been extracted and the model has been chosen, the next step is to train the model on a data set. During this process, the model's parameters are adjusted to minimize the error between the model's predictions and true value. The success of an ML model is usually evaluated in three categories: performance, resources required, and prediction accuracy [56]. Of these three, accuracy is perhaps the most important and difficult metric to assess because it requires an additional independent test dataset. The test dataset is given to the ML model and the predictions are compared against the true value or ground truth. If the model's performance is not satisfactory, it may be necessary to fine-tune the model by adjusting its hyperparameters or by training the model on additional data sets. Once the model has been trained and evaluated, it can be deployed to make predictions on new, unseen data.

5.2.2 Using machine learning for optical coherence tomography angiography analysis

Recently, ML image analysis methods have become an area of interest in OCTA research. Specifically, researchers aim to use AI to accurately detect pathology, precisely quantify retinal vasculature, and reliably diagnose disease [58]. In 2019, Chan et al. used features of the ONH and retina to automatically diagnose glaucoma from macular and disk images [59]. In this pilot study, the authors used the AdaBoost Classifier model, a self-adjusting classification tool. They reported excellent model accuracy of 94.3% on 109 images (57 normal, 52 glaucoma). This milestone study showed that ML could aid clinicians in glaucoma detection at an early stage.

In 2022, Kooner et al. developed an ML tool to identify the parameters which provided the most accurate diagnosis of glaucoma [60]. The authors analyzed six ML algorithms, and over 2500 ML models were optimized using random search. In this study, the XGBoost algorithm, a highly effective and scalable ML model, achieved the highest accuracy of 83.9%. They also explored the ML decision tree models to understand the most useful diagnostic parameters (inferior temporal VD, inferior hemisphere VD, and peripapillary RNFL thickness).

5.2.3 Overview of deep learning methodology

DL is a subset of ML which uses artificial networks composed of "neurons" or nodes layered to resemble the human brain. DL algorithms can understand complex patterns and relationships in the data by adjusting the weights and biases of the connections between the neurons in the network. While DL architectures are more powerful learners than ML algorithms, they are less customizable and interpretable [56]. Additionally, DL models are very practical since they are able to automatically extract features from raw input data resulting in increased efficiency and pattern recognition. Convolutional neural networks (CNNs), a type of DL architecture specialized for image input data, are particularly useful for extracting features for DL training. They operate in a bottom-up manner, first identifying basic features such as corners and working up towards more complex structures. Similar performance metrics are utilized for both ML and DL models.

A disadvantage of DL is the need for a large volume of clinical data during the training process. This data acquisition process can be affected by privacy concerns and time constraints. DL tools which can be used to address this need for data are known as generative adversarial networks (GANs). GANs are a type of DL algorithm that are used for generating new, synthetic data that is similar to a given dataset. GANs are composed of two neural networks: a generator network, which is responsible for generating new data, and a discriminator network, which can distinguish the synthetic and real data. The goal of GANs is to generate synthetic data that is indistinguishable from real data, addressing issues posed in conventional data acquisition processes.

5.2.4 Using deep learning for optical coherence tomography angiography analysis

In recent years, the use of CNNs for automated glaucoma diagnosis has grown in popularity over prior ML techniques. In 2022, Bowd et al. used CNNs to improve the performance of feature-based gradient boosting classifier (GBC) analysis, an ML technique that combines multiple subsets of models to create a powerful classification tool, in 405 images (130 healthy, 275 glaucoma) [61]. GBC models were separately trained on OCT and OCTA scans of the ONH, while the CNN model was trained solely on region proposal classifier (RPC), a type of DL architecture used for object detection tasks. To account for the imbalance of healthy and glaucomatous eyes, areas under the precision recall curves (AUPRC) were computed to evaluate the performance of the two models. The CNN model had an AUPRC of 0.97, compared 0.93 for the best ML model, indicating that the DL models improve on feature-based ML models for classifying healthy and glaucomatous eyes.

In 2022 Kumar et al. used GANs to create synthetic OCT circumpapillary images, evaluate them for gradeability and authenticity, and use them to train DL models [62]. The researchers created two models to generate both healthy and glaucomatous synthetic OCT images of the circumpapillary ONH. The optimal DL network trained on synthetic images (AUC = 0.97 internal test data vs. 0.90 external test data), while the DL network trained with real images performed worse (AUC = 0.96 internal test data vs. 0.84 external test data). The accuracy of DL networks trained with synthetic images were comparable to those trained with real images, indicating their potential use for other modalities such as OCTA and similar DL applications.

DL can also be used to enhance the quality of OCT and OCTA images affected by artifacts and speckle noise (noise caused by the coherent scattering of the light waves used to acquire the image). Early studies by Yamashita et al. used modified CNN tools to enhance the scan quality of noisy ONH OCTs [63]. Recently, Omodoka et al. denoised RPC OCTA images to improve the quality of calculated RPC vessel area density and vessel length density [64].

Since DL automated feature extraction acts like a "black box" concept, studies explaining DL decision making are vital. These "explainability" studies attempt to address the interpretability of DL, which will be crucial for clinical implementation. To better understand DL decision making, Hemelings et al. conducted a study on fundus images to determine the importance of the regions outside of the ONH for DL-based glaucoma detection and vertical CDR (VCDR) [65]. The researchers trained DL models on a database of 23,930 images and compared classification accuracy. They showed that models trained on the original unaltered images (AUC = 0.94, VCDR estimation = 77%) outperformed models that were trained on images with the absence of the ONH (AUC =0.80, VCDR estimation = 37%). Thus, these results provide evidence that DL models that use areas beyond the ONH, such as VCDR, are superior in classifying glaucomatous eyes.

6. Conclusion

Since the introduction of OCTA concept, the technology has increased the understanding of both the structural and vascular damage seen in patients with glaucoma. Not only is OCTA a safe, non-invasive, and quick test it provides the same structural information as OCT such as retinal and RNFL thinning, but it can also visualize relevant vascular parameters such as ONH VD and macular VD that typically undergo glaucomatous damage. However, significant limitations of OCTA such as a high prevalence of artifacts and lack of standardization across different machines currently do exist and must be accounted for while using this technology. Despite these limitations, the advantages of being able to observe both the structural and vascular damage caused by glaucoma show why OCTA is currently being adopted by ophthalmologists. In addition, the progress made in incorporating ML and DL techniques with OCTA will aid both in the diagnosis and progression in glaucoma.

Terminology

Disk perfusion: Refers to flow index and vessel density of the disk region.

Flow index: Average decorrelation values provided by the SSADA algorithm.

Focal loss volume (%): Describes the average focal loss of ganglion cells in the ganglion cell complex layer of the retina.

Global loss volume (%): Describes the average overall loss of ganglion cells in the ganglion cell complex of the retina.

Vessel density (%): Area occupied by blood vessels in any particular segment of the retina or ONH.

Vessel length density (%): Length of the vasculature divided by total image area.

Acknowledgements

This study was supported in part by NIH core grant P30 EY030413 (Bethesda, Maryland), NIH award UL1TR001105 (Bethesda, Maryland), and University of Texas Southwestern Medical Student Research Program (Dallas, TX). The content is solely the responsibility of the authors and does not necessarily represent the official views of the NIH. We would also like to thank Tina Pham, Priya Mekala, and Monica Patel for their help with organizing artifact images and information.

Abbreviations

AI	Artificial intelligence
AUC	Area under the curve
AUPRC	Areas under the precision recall curves
AUROC	Area under receiver operator characteristic curve
CCT	Central corneal thickness
CDR	Cup/disk ratio
CNN	Convolutional neural network
CV	Coefficient of variation
DL	Deep learning
FAZ	Foveal avascular zone
GAN	Generative adversarial network
IOP	Intraocular pressure
LPQ	Local phase quantization
mGCC	Macular ganglion cell complex
ML	Machine learning
MVD	Microvascular dropout
NFL	Nerve fiber layer
OCT	Optical coherence tomography
OCTA	Optical coherence tomography angiography
OMAG	Optical microangiography
ONH	Optic nerve head
PCA	Principal component analysis
POAG	Primary open angle glaucoma
PPG	Preperimetric glaucoma
PXG	Pseudoexfoliative glaucoma
RGC	Retinal ganglion cell
RNFL	Retinal nerve fiber layer
RPC	Region proposal classifier
SSADA	Split-spectrum amplitude decorrelation angiography
SSI	Signal strength intensity
SVC	Superficial vascular complex
VCDR	Vertical cup/disk ratio
VD	Vessel density
VF	Visual field
VFMS	Visual field mean sensitivity

Author details

Karanjit Kooner[1,2*], Mahad Rehman[1], Sruthi Suresh[1], Emily Buchanan[1], Mohannad Albdour[3] and Hafsa Zuberi[1]

1 Department of Ophthalmology, The University of Texas Southwestern Medical Center, Dallas, Texas, USA

2 Veterans Affairs, North Texas Healthcare System, Dallas, Texas, USA

3 Department of Ophthalmology, King Hussein Medical Center, Amman, Jordan

*Address all correspondence to: karanjit.kooner@utsouthwestern.edu

References

[1] Tham YC, Li X, Wong TY, Quigley HA, Aung T, Cheng CY. Global prevalence of glaucoma and projections of glaucoma burden through 2040: A systematic review and meta-analysis. Ophthalmology. 2014;**121**(11):2081-2090

[2] Gedde SJ, Vinod K, Wright MM, Muir KW, Lind JT, Chen PP, et al. Primary open-angle glaucoma preferred practice pattern®. Ophthalmology. 2021;**128**(1):71-150

[3] Müller H. Anatomische Beiträge zur Ophthalmologie. Archiv für Ophthalmologie. 1858;**4**(2):1-54

[4] Jaeger RV, Eduard J. Über Glaukom und seine Heilung durch Iridektomie. Z Ges Aerzte Wien. 1858;**30**:465-484

[5] Bussel II, Wollstein G, Schuman JS. OCT for glaucoma diagnosis, screening, and detection of glaucoma progression. Br J Ophthalmol. 2014;**98**(Suppl. 2): ii15-ii19

[6] Spaide RF, Fujimoto JG, Waheed NK. Optical coherence tomography angiography. Retina. 2015;**35**(11): 2161-2162

[7] KumarRS,AnegondiN,ChandapuraRS, Sudhakaran S, Kadambi SV, Rao HL, et al. Discriminant function of optical coherence tomography angiography to determine disease severity in glaucoma. Investigative Ophthalmology & Visual Science. 2016;**57**(14):6079-6088

[8] Yarmohammadi A, Zangwill LM, Diniz-Filho A, Suh MH, Manalastas PI, Fatehee N, et al. Optical coherence tomography angiography vessel density in healthy, glaucoma suspect, and glaucoma eyes. Invest Ophthalmol Vis Sci. 2016;**57**(9):451-459

[9] AlSalem M, Yang A, Noorani S, Deng T, Li X, Adams-Huet B, et al. Effectiveness of optical coherence tomography angiography (OCT-A) in staging glaucoma. Journal of the Royal Medical Services. 2022;**29**(2):1-15

[10] Huang D, Swanson EA, Lin CP, Schuman JS, Stinson WG, Chang W, et al. Optical coherence tomography. Science. 1991;**254**(5035):1178-1181

[11] Fujimoto J, Swanson E. The development, commercialization, and impact of optical coherence tomography. Invest Ophthalmol Vis Sci. 2016;**57**(9):Oct1-oct13

[12] Optovue Receives FDA. Clearance for Cornea/Anterior Module for RTVue. Company Website; 2006

[13] Fercher AF, Hitzenberger CK, Kamp G, El-Zaiat SY. Measurement of intraocular distances by backscattering spectral interferometry. Optics Communications. 1995;**117**(1):43-48

[14] White B, Pierce M, Nassif N, Cense B, Park B, Tearney G, et al. In vivo dynamic human retinal blood flow imaging using ultra-high-speed spectral domain optical coherence tomography. Optics Express. 2003;**11**(25):3490-3497

[15] Zhang J, Chen Z. In vivo blood flow imaging by a swept laser source-based Fourier domain optical Doppler tomography. Optics Express. 2005;**13**(19):7449-7457

[16] Spaide RF, Koizumi H, Pozzoni MC. Enhanced depth imaging spectral-domain optical coherence tomography. American Journal of Ophthalmology. 2008;**146**(4):496-500

[17] Walsh AC. Binocular optical coherence tomography. Ophthalmic Surgery, Lasers & Imaging. 2011;**42**(Suppl):S95-s105

[18] Jia Y, Tan O, Tokayer J, Potsaid B, Wang Y, Liu JJ, et al. Split-spectrum amplitude-decorrelation angiography with optical coherence tomography. Optics Express. 2012;**20**(4):4710-4725

[19] Reif R, Qin J, An L, Zhi Z, Dziennis S, Wang R. Quantifying optical microangiography images obtained from a spectral domain optical coherence tomography system. International Journal of Biomedical Imaging. 2012;**2012**:509783

[20] Choi W, Mohler KJ, Potsaid B, Lu CD, Liu JJ, Jayaraman V, et al. Choriocapillaris and choroidal microvasculature imaging with ultrahigh speed OCT angiography. PLoS One. 2013;**8**(12):e81499

[21] Spaide RF, Fujimoto JG, Waheed NK, Sadda SR, Staurenghi G. Optical coherence tomography angiography. Progress in Retinal and Eye Research. 2018;**64**:1-55

[22] Zhang A, Zhang Q, Wang RK. Minimizing projection artifacts for accurate presentation of choroidal neovascularization in OCT micro-angiography. Biomedical Optics Express. 2015;**6**(10):4130-4143

[23] Liu L, Gao SS, Bailey ST, Huang D, Li D, Jia Y. Automated choroidal neovascularization detection algorithm for optical coherence tomography angiography. Biomedical Optics Express. 2015;**6**(9):3564-3576

[24] Yoshikawa YST, Kanno J, Kimura I, Hangai M, Shinoda K. Optic disc vessel density in nonglaucomatous and glaucomatous eyes: An enhanced-depth imaging optical coherence tomography angiography study. Clinical Ophthalmology. 2018;**12**:1113-1119

[25] Le PH, Patel BC. Optical Coherence Tomography Angiography. Treasure Island (FL): StatPearls; 2022

[26] Browning DJ, Glassman AR, Aiello LP, Bressler NM, Bressler SB, Danis RP, et al. Optical coherence tomography measurements and analysis methods in optical coherence tomography studies of diabetic macular edema. Ophthalmology. 2008;**115**(8):1366-1371, 71.e1

[27] Bhende M, Shetty S, Parthasarathy M, Ramya S. Optical coherence tomography: A guide to interpretation of common macular diseases. Indian Journal of Ophthalmology. 2018;**66**(1):20-35

[28] Nesper PL, Fawzi AA. Human Parafoveal capillary vascular anatomy and connectivity revealed by optical coherence tomography angiography. Investigative Ophthalmology & Visual Science. 2018;**59**(10):3858-3867

[29] Jia Y, Wei E, Wang X, Zhang X, Morrison JC, Parikh M, et al. Optical coherence tomography angiography of optic disc perfusion in glaucoma. Ophthalmology. 2014;**121**(7):1322-1332

[30] Chen CL, Bojikian KD, Gupta D, Wen JC, Zhang Q, Xin C, et al. Optic nerve head perfusion in normal eyes and eyes with glaucoma using optical coherence tomography-based microangiography. Quantitative Imaging in Medicine and Surgery. 2016;**6**(2):125-133

[31] Andrade De Jesus D, Sánchez Brea L, Barbosa Breda J, Fokkinga E, Ederveen V, Borren N, et al. OCTA multilayer and multisector Peripapillary microvascular modeling for diagnosing and staging of

glaucoma. Translational Vision Science & Technology. 2020;**9**(2):58

[32] Bekkers A, Borren N, Ederveen V, Fokkinga E. Andrade De Jesus D, Sánchez Brea L, et al. microvascular damage assessed by optical coherence tomography angiography for glaucoma diagnosis: A systematic review of the most discriminative regions. Acta Ophthalmologica. 2020;**98**(6):537-558

[33] Eslami Y, Ghods S, Mohammadi M, Safizadeh M, Fakhraie G, Zarei R, et al. The role of optical coherence tomography angiography in moderate and advanced primary open-angle glaucoma. International Ophthalmology. 2022;**42**(12):3645-3659

[34] Mohammadzadeh V, Fatehi N, Yarmohammadi A, Lee JW, Sharifipour F, Daneshvar R, et al. Macular imaging with optical coherence tomography in glaucoma. Survey of Ophthalmology. 2020;**65**(6):597-638

[35] Takusagawa HL, Liu L, Ma KN, Jia Y, Gao SS, Zhang M, et al. Projection-resolved optical coherence tomography angiography of macular retinal circulation in glaucoma. Ophthalmology. 2017;**124**(11):1589-1599

[36] Kim J-A, Lee EJ, Kim T-W. Evaluation of parapapillary choroidal microvasculature dropout and progressive retinal nerve fiber layer thinning in patients with glaucoma. JAMA Ophthalmology. 2019;**137**(7):810-816

[37] Chatziralli I, Milionis I, ChristodoulouA,TheodossiadisP,KitsosG. The role of vessel density as measured by optical coherence tomography angiography in the evaluation of Pseudoexfoliative glaucoma: A review of the literature. Ophthalmol Ther. 2022;**11**(2):533-545

[38] Chen HS, Liu CH, Wu WC, Tseng HJ, Lee YS. Optical coherence tomography angiography of the superficial microvasculature in the macular and Peripapillary areas in glaucomatous and healthy eyes. Investigative Ophthalmology & Visual Science. 2017;**58**(9):3637-3645

[39] Geyman LS, Garg RA, Suwan Y, Trivedi V, Krawitz BD, Mo S, et al. Peripapillary perfused capillary density in primary open-angle glaucoma across disease stage: An optical coherence tomography angiography study. The British Journal of Ophthalmology. 2017;**101**(9):1261-1268

[40] Bowd C, Belghith A, Rezapour J, Christopher M, Hyman L, Jonas JB, et al. Diagnostic accuracy of macular thickness map and texture En face images for detecting glaucoma in eyes with axial high myopia. American Journal of Ophthalmology. 2022;**242**:26-35

[41] Suwan Y, Fard MA, Geyman LS, Tantraworasin A, Chui TY, Rosen RB, et al. Association of Myopia with Peripapillary perfused capillary density in patients with glaucoma: An optical coherence tomography angiography study. JAMA Ophthalmology. 2018;**136**(5):507-513

[42] Chang PY, Wang JY, Wang JK, Huang TL, Hsu YR. Optical coherence tomography angiography compared with optical coherence tomography for detection of early glaucoma with high myopia. Front Med (Lausanne). 2021;**8**:793786

[43] Shin JW, Kwon J, Lee J, et al. Relationship between vessel density and visual field sensitivity in glaucomatous eyes with high myopia. The British Journal of Ophthalmology. 2019;**103**:585-591

[44] Yilmaz H, Yeşiltaş YS, Aydemir E, Aksoy Aydemir G, Gökgöz Özışık G,

Koylu MT, et al. A myopic normative database for retinal nerve fiber layer thickness using optical coherence tomography. Journal of Glaucoma. 2022;**31**(10):816-825

[45] Protsyk O, Gallego-Pinazo R, Dolz-Marco R. Limitaciones actuales y futuro de la angiografía por tomografía de coherencia óptica. Archivos de la Sociedad Española de Oftalmología. 2022;**97**(8):421-423

[46] Anvari P, Ashrafkhorasani M, Habibi A, Falavarjani KG. Artifacts in optical coherence tomography angiography. J. Ophthalmic Vis. Res. 2021;**16**(2):271-286

[47] Kamalipour A, Moghimi S, Hou H, Penteado RC, Oh WH, Proudfoot JA, et al. OCT angiography artifacts in glaucoma. Ophthalmology. 2021;**128**(10):1426-1437

[48] Cheng W, Song Y, Lin F, Xiong J, Li F, Jin L, et al. Assessment of artifacts in swept-source optical coherence tomography angiography for glaucomatous and Normal eyes. Translational Vision Science & Technology. 2022;**11**(1):23

[49] PKP M, Patel M, Kim-Cavdar KKS, editors. OCT-A artifacts in healthy, ocular hypertension, glaucoma suspect, myopic and glaucomatous eyes. In: American Academy of Ophthalmology Annual Meeting. Chicago, IL; 2022

[50] Weijing C, Zhang X, Wang W. Artifacts associated with swept-source OCT-angiography measurements in glaucoma. Investigative Ophthalmology & Visual Science. 2020;**61**(7):4117

[51] Ferguson RD, Hammer DX, Paunescu LA, Beaton S, Schuman JS. Tracking optical coherence tomography. Optics Letters. 2004;**29**(18):2139-2141

[52] Venugopal JP, Rao HL, Weinreb RN, Dasari S, Riyazuddin M, Pradhan ZS, et al. Repeatability and comparability of peripapillary vessel density measurements of high-density and non-high-density optical coherence tomography angiography scans in normal and glaucoma eyes. The British Journal of Ophthalmology. 2019;**103**(7):949-954

[53] Manalastas PIC, Zangwill LM, Saunders LJ, Mansouri K, Belghith A, Suh MH, et al. Reproducibility of optical coherence tomography angiography macular and optic nerve head vascular density in glaucoma and healthy eyes. Journal of Glaucoma. 2017;**26**(10):851-859

[54] Munk MR, Kashani AH, Tadayoni R, Korobelnik JF, Wolf S, Pichi F, et al. Standardization of OCT angiography nomenclature in retinal vascular diseases: First survey results. Ophthalmol Retina. 2021;**5**(10):981-990

[55] Sampson DM, Dubis AM, Chen FK, Zawadzki RJ, Sampson DD. Towards standardizing retinal optical coherence tomography angiography: A review. Light: Science & Applications. 2022;**11**(1):63

[56] Janiesch C, Zschech P, Heinrich K. Machine learning and deep learning. Electronic Markets. 2021;**31**(3):685-695

[57] Le D, Son T, Yao X. Machine learning in optical coherence tomography angiography. Experimental Biology and Medicine (Maywood, N.J.). 2021;**246**(20):2170-2183

[58] Hormel TT, Hwang TS, Bailey ST, Wilson DJ, Huang D, Jia Y. Artificial intelligence in OCT angiography. Progress in Retinal and Eye Research. 2021;**85**:100965

[59] Chan YM, Ng EYK, Jahmunah V, Wei Koh JE, Lih OS, Wei Leon LY, et al.

Automated detection of glaucoma using optical coherence tomography angiogram images. Computers in Biology and Medicine. 2019;**115**:103483

[60] Kooner KS, Angirekula A, TreacherAH,Al-HumimatG,MarzbanMF, Chen A, et al. Glaucoma diagnosis through the integration of optical coherence tomography/angiography and machine learning diagnostic models. Clinical Ophthalmology. 2022;**16**:2685-2697

[61] Bowd C, Belghith A, Zangwill LM, Christopher M, Goldbaum MH, Fan R, et al. Deep learning image analysis of optical coherence tomography angiography measured vessel density improves classification of healthy and glaucoma eyes. American Journal of Ophthalmology. 2022;**236**:298-308

[62] Sreejith Kumar AJ, Chong RS, Crowston JG, Chua J, Bujor I, Husain R, et al. Evaluation of generative adversarial networks for high-resolution synthetic image generation of Circumpapillary optical coherence tomography images for glaucoma. JAMA Ophthalmol. 2022;**140**(10):974-981

[63] Yamashita K, Markov K, editors. Medical image enhancement using super resolution methods. In: Computational Science–ICCS 2020. Cham: Springer International Publishing;

[64] Omodaka K, Horie J, Tokairin H, Kato C, Ouchi J, Ninomiya T, et al. Deep learning-based noise reduction improves optical coherence tomography angiography imaging of radial Peripapillary capillaries in advanced glaucoma. Current Eye Research. 2022;**47**(12):1600-1608

[65] Hemelings R, Elen B, Barbosa-Breda J, Blaschko MB, De Boever P, Stalmans I. Deep learning on fundus images detects glaucoma beyond the optic disc. Scientific Reports. 2021;**11**(1):20313

Chapter 6

Morphofunctional Changes of the Retina and Optic Nerve in Optical Neuropathy of Various Genesis: A Literature Review

Svetlana Zhukova, Tatiana Iureva and Dmitry Samsonov

Abstract

The retina is part of the central nervous system and has much in common with the brain's physiological characteristics. Ophthalmological manifestations often precede the symptoms of central nervous system disorders and are used for their early diagnosis. Retinal imaging is simpler and more economical than the available central nervous system imaging methods. In this connection, the search for retinal biomarkers of neurodegenerative diseases is relevant. Optical coherence tomography is highly valuable both for routine clinical practice and for research purposes. Different patterns of structural changes of the optic nerve and retina in optical neuropathies of various genesis are due to differences in the pathogenesis of diseases (glaucoma optic neuropathy, non-arterial anterior ischemic optic neuropathy, optic neuritis associated with multiple sclerosis, and compression optic neuropathy). The identified biomarkers can be used for screening patients in primary healthcare institutions to provide a preliminary diagnosis of patients at risk.

Keywords: optical coherence tomography (OCT), optical coherence tomography angiography (OCTA), ganglion cells complex (GCC), retinal nerve fibers layer (RNFL), optic nerve, neurodegenerative diseases

1. Introduction

In the general cascade of events leading to irreversible changes in the optic nerve, damage to the nerve fiber layer, and the retinal ganglion cell complex (GCC) are important factors contributing to the optical neuropathy pathogenesis of any genesis [1–7]. The possibility of retrograde trans-synaptic degeneration of visual fibers in visual pathway central neuron damage [8] opens up new prospects for visualizing morphological changes in the central nervous system (CNS) at the retinal level, since the retina being a part of the central nervous system, has much in common with the physiological characteristics of the brain.

The organization of visual pathway neural links is quite complex. Within the retina of every eye, it is a layer of photoreceptors (I neuron), then bipolar (II neuron)

and ganglion cells with their long axons (III neuron). Together, they form the peripheral part of the visual pathway, represented by the optic nerves, chiasm and visual tracts. The visual tracts end in the cells of the corpus geniculatum laterale (CGL), which is the primary visual center. Central neuron fibers of the visual pathway (radiatio optica Gratiolet) originate from them and reach the area striate of the occipital lobe of the brain, where the primary cortical center of the visual analyzer is localized (**Figure 1**) [9].

The uniqueness of the visual pathway organization is that there is only one synapse between the retina and the visual cortex. Thus, any damage to the optic nerve head (ONH) will lead to trans-synaptic (trans-neuronal) degeneration in both anterograde and retrograde directions. Trans-synaptic anterograde degeneration leads to changes in the CGL, radiatio optica, and visual cortex, and trans-synaptic retrograde degeneration leads to changes in the retinal ganglion cell complex (GCC) (**Figure 1**) [10, 11].

Ophthalmoscopic manifestations of neurodegenerative diseases often precede the symptoms of CNS disorders and are used for their diagnosis. In turn, retinal visualization is much simpler and more economical than the available methods of CNS visualization.

The most technologically advanced and dynamically developing imaging method in ophthalmology is optical coherence tomography (OCT). Qualitative assessment

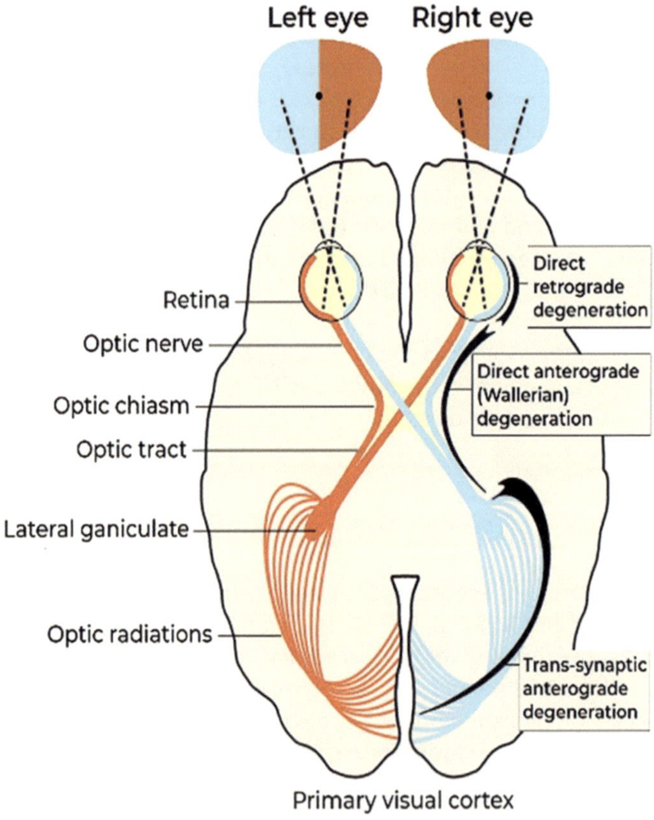

Figure 1.
The structure of the visual pathway.

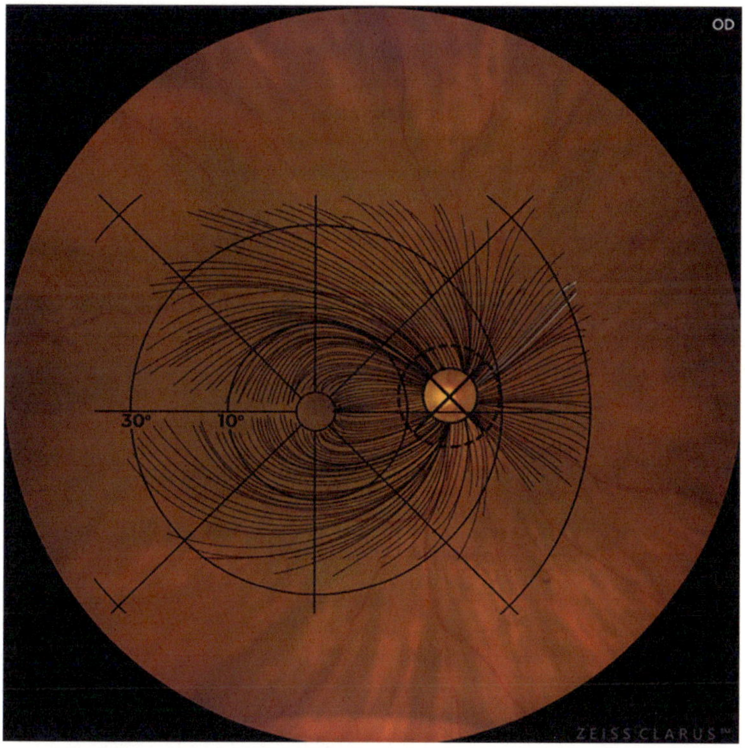

Figure 2.
Retinal nerve fiber layer topography.

and quantitative analysis, integrated into the tomography software, allow identifying pathological changes in the studied structures with high repeatability and specificity.

When evaluating OCT images, it is necessary to understand the factors that determine the structural changes' range. The topography of the retinal nerve fibers layer (RNFL) is characterized by strict regularity. Ganglion cell axons extending from the central retinal region, as a part of the papillomacular bundle, form the temporal part of the ONH. Fibers extending from the superior-temporal and inferior-temporal retinal quadrants form the superior-temporal and inferior-temporal segments, respectively. Axons extending from ganglion cells located nasally and along the retinal periphery penetrate into the optic nerve disc from the nasal side. From the periphery of the temporal part of the retina, axons are directed to the superior and inferior parts of the ONH (**Figure 2**) [12].

Various patterns of damage to the RNFL and GCC are caused by the pathogenesis of neurons' primary damage. These differences can be used as differential diagnostic criteria for glaucomatous and non-glaucomatous optical neuropathies in routine clinical practice.

2. Glaucoma optic neuropathy

Primary open-angle glaucoma is a chronic progressive optical neuropathy resulting from damage to retinal ganglion cells [13, 14]. Damage to the GCC axons in glaucoma is initialized in the optic nerve head by various mechanisms, such as mechanical compression of intraocular pressure, vascular disorders, immunological influence, and oxidative stress. This can lead to direct retrograde damage to the GCC, followed by thinning of the RNFL and visual field defects [15].

A comprehensive assessment of early-onset glaucoma and its subsequent monitoring is achieved by combining the results of "structure-function." The key diagnostic methods for glaucoma are OCT and static automated perimetry (SAP). Each of the methods has its advantages and limitations.

Structural and functional relationships reach their peak at the advanced stage of the disease [16]. At early and late stages of glaucoma, there may be contradictions between OCT and SAP [17–20].

OCT allows for obtaining objective information about the retinal layers' thickness with high repeatability and reproducibility. Diagnostic OCT markers of POAG are the width of the rim area, RNFL, and GCC thickness [21, 22].

The temporal half of the superior and inferior quadrants of the optic nerve head are the most vulnerable areas of peripapillary RNFL loss—the superior and inferior vulnerable zones (superior vulnerable zone—SVZ & inferior vulnerable zone—IVZ) [23–25]. In severe glaucoma, the values reach a "floor effect" level [26].

With the progression of glaucoma, the defects area increases. With a decrease in the thickness of the RNFL and GCC to the "floor" level (50–70% of the nerve fiber layer thickness of healthy eyes), the existence of functional axons in the remaining layer is assumed, but the total number of these axons does not significantly contribute to the thickness of the layer [16, 27].

Nevertheless, the papillomacular bundle and high central vision in glaucoma patients persist until the later stages of the disease. The inferior macular zone associated with arcuate defects of peripapillary nerve fibers is more vulnerable, therefore, in the late stage of the disease, asymmetric preservation of the macula is often observed.

At the same time, in early glaucoma, SAP may not be informative, because statistically significant visual field defects are detected with 25–35% loss of retinal ganglion cells [28]. Visual field defects are not detected in the early stages due to the inability of the SAP to detect small functional losses as a result of the redundancy of the visual system and the overlap of receptive fields [29]. In addition, the SAP method is subjective, high concentration is required from the patient during the study, which can reduce the repeatability and reproducibility of testing.

The software of modern computer perimeters provides wide opportunities for analyzing threshold values of retinal photosensitivity. Thus, sensitivity to early glaucoma changes increases with cluster analysis, when the test points of the visual field are located and grouped along the course of a single bundle of retinal nerve fibers (clusters). The mean cluster photosensitivity defect is calculated for every cluster (**Figure 3**) [30, 31].

In addition to cluster analysis, anatomically oriented polar analysis is carried out in the Octopus perimeter [32]. It provides information about the expected location of morphological lesions of the rim area in the optic nerve head. Each visual field defect is combined with a nerve fibers bundle that hypothetically corresponds to it. Then, a vector is applied to the diagram of the optic nerve head at a certain angle corresponding to the localization of the defect, the length of which reflects the loss of photosensitivity in dB (**Figure 3**).

The addition of central test points to Protocol 24-2, 30-2, and macular area testing (Protocol 10-2) increases the effectiveness of testing [33].

To compare structural and functional defects, RNFL and GCC thickness maps can be superimposed on the test points of the visual field (24-2 location on the FNFL thickness map and 10-2 on the GCC thickness maps) (**Figure 4**).

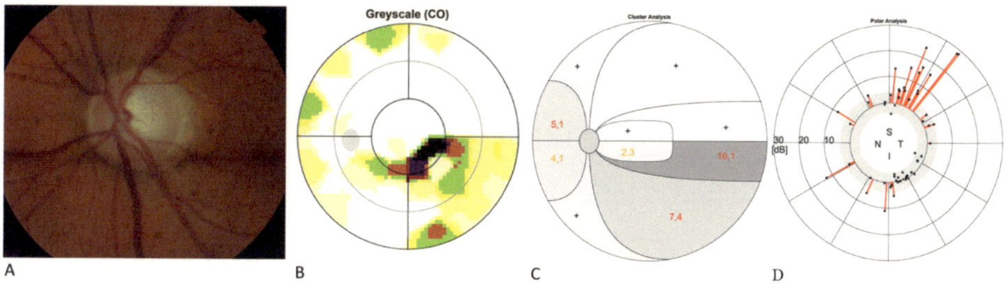

Figure 3.
54-year-old man with glaucoma. A—fundus-image. B—grayscale of values. The color scale indicates the absolute values of the light sensitivity thresholds in the form of a color map. C—cluster analysis. The degree of background darkening reflects the degree of deviation of clusters from the norm. D—polar analysis. The gray sector is in the normal range. The red vector is the radial coordinate. The length of the vector indicates the length of the defect. The angular coordinate is determined by the entry angle of nerve fibers bundles connected to each test point in the optic nerve disk.

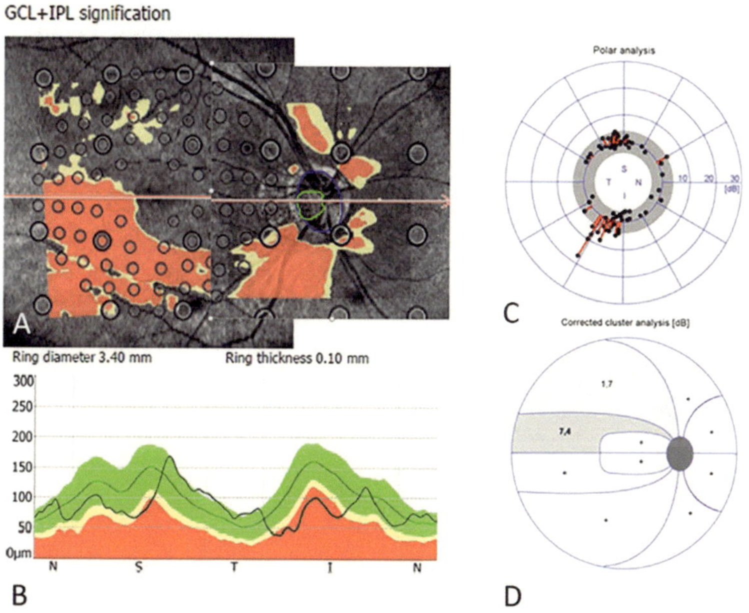

Figure 4.
Spatial correspondence of structural-functional indicators. A 48-year-old man with glaucoma. BCVA 1.0. A—superposition of abnormal points of the visual field on RNFL and GCC probability maps (Revo NX, Optopol). B—NSTIN-RNFL profile color-coded. C—polar analysis. D—cluster analysis.

A better understanding of the spatial correspondence of structural-functional indicators is facilitated by the representation of the profile of the peripapillary nerve fibers layer in the form of a scan graph NSTIN (nasal, N; superior, S; temporal, T; inferior, I; nasal, N), when the indicators of the RNFL thickness from the temporal half of the disk are presented in the middle of the graph (**Figure 4**) [34].

The evolution of OCT in ophthalmology has led to the emergence of a fundamentally new research method—OCT angiography (OCTA). OCTA is a new method of noninvasive visualization of blood vessels in the ONH and retina *in vivo* [35, 36].

Localized RNFL defects are spatially associated with density reduction of peripapillary vessels, even in early and preperimetric glaucoma. The most pronounced differences in OCTA indices between groups of healthy individuals and glaucoma patients were found in the inferior-temporal and superior-temporal quadrants of the peripapillary retina. Thus, the relationship between structural and functional, and hemodynamic changes in patients with POAG is obvious (**Figure 5**) [37, 38].

At the same time, multifunctional correlations are stronger than structural-functional ones [39].

Thus, the OCTA method is promising and, along with structural OCT and visual field testing, can become part of everyday routine practice. Today, OCTA is successfully used in the primary diagnosis of glaucoma, differential diagnosis of glaucoma in combined pathology, disease monitoring, and hemodynamic shifts assessment in IOP fluctuations [40, 41].

The characteristic pattern of RNFL and GCC damage in glaucoma is asymmetric paracentral macular defects associated with arcuate defects of the peripapillary RNFL, corresponding to them a density reduction of the peripapillary and parafoveolar capillaries, and perimetric defects.

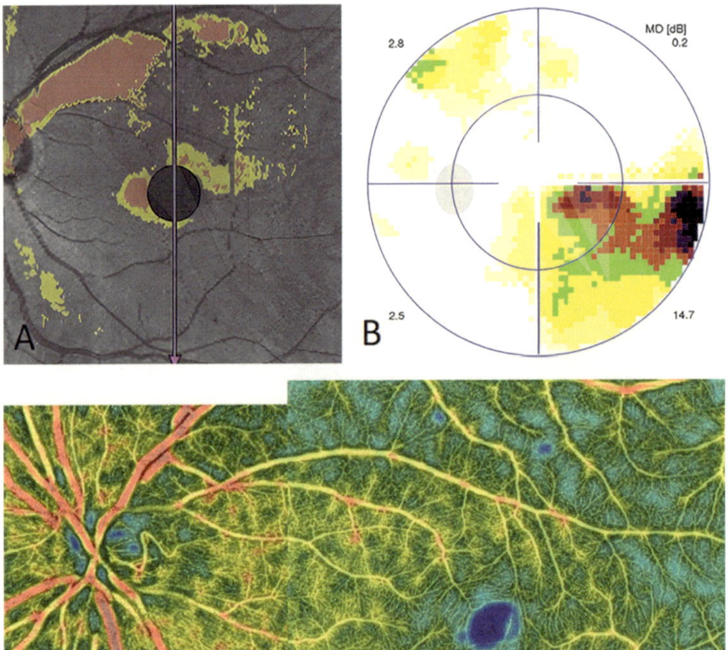

Figure 5.
54-year-old man with advanced glaucoma. BCVA 1.0. A—OCT probability map of RNFL and GCC. B—grayscale of values. C—OCTA, capillary density of the radial peripapillary plexus and the superficial plexus. A significant decrease in the peripapillary and parafoveolar capillaries density, corresponds to the thinning of GCC and RNFL.

3. Non-arterial anterior ischemic optic neuropathy

Non-arterial anterior ischemic optic neuropathy (NAION) is the second most common optical neuropathy after glaucoma optic neuropathy (GON) among middle-aged and older people caused by hypoperfusion in the posterior short ciliary arteries that supply blood to the ONH [42–44].

The pathogenesis of NATION is not fully known. However, anatomical predisposition, narrow scleral canal, optic disc druses, systemic hypertension, diabetes mellitus, cardiovascular diseases, and hypercholesterolemia are risk factors for NAION [45]. Ischemic damage to the optic nerve head triggers a vicious circle of increasing ischemia. Hypoxia of axons of ganglion cells blocks axoplasmic current and leads to edema of the ONH. The optic nerve is quite rigid, so axons can expand only due to the compression of surrounding tissues (the mechanism of compartment syndrome). Compression of capillaries and smaller vessels increases axonal hypoperfusion, which, in turn, leads to further axoplasmic stagnation and edema [46, 47].

Diagnosis of NAION in the acute phase with painless loss of vision for several hours or days, ONH edema does not cause difficulties. In the chronic stage, it can be

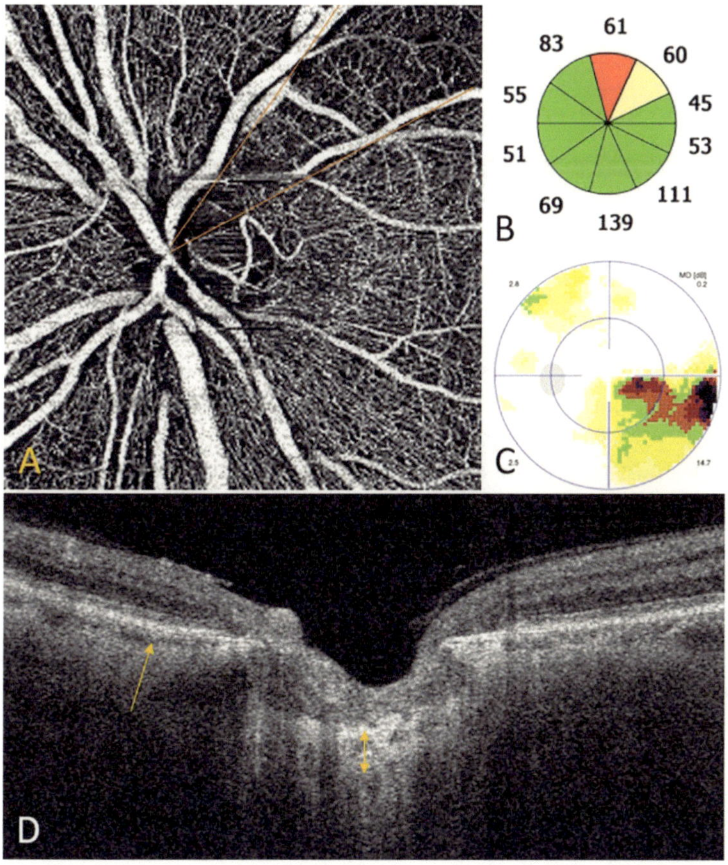

Figure 6.
48-year-old man with GON. A—OCTA, radial peripapillary plexus, B—a graph of RFNL thickness, C—grayscale of values, D—ONH b-scan and peripapillary retina.

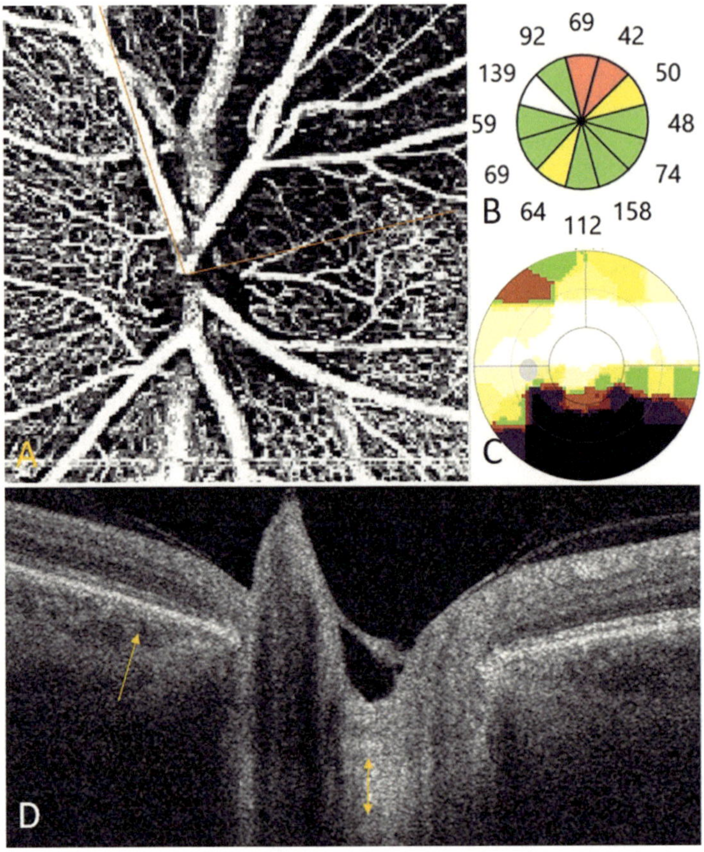

Figure 7.
42-year-old man with NAION. A—OCTA, radial peripapillary plexus, B—a graph of RFNL thickness, C—grayscale of values, D—ONH b-scan and peripapillary retina.

difficult to differentiate NAION from GON, since the pattern of RNFL loss and visual field defects may be similar (**Figures 6** and 7).

Despite the comparable thickness of the nerve fiber layer in both patients, a patient with NAON has a more diffuse decrease in peripapillary capillaries and a more pronounced depression of the visual field, a greater thickness of the peripapillary choroid and the lamina cribrosa.

The importance of differential diagnosis is due to different prognosis and treatment approaches. There are no effective methods of NAION therapy. Treatment is reduced to the elimination of vascular risk factors to prevent the occurrence of the disease in the paired eye [48]. Therefore, a correct diagnosis will prevent unnecessary excessive treatment that is prescribed due to incorrect diagnosis of NAION as glaucoma.

Similar to glaucoma, NAION also leads to the loss of ganglion cells and damage to the RNFL in the superior and inferior quadrants. However, in contrast to GON, in NAION the damage to the RNFL in the superior and inferior quadrants is more diffuse (from the temporal to the nasal edge) (**Figure 7**). Defects of the RNFL in the superior quadrant are formed more often. The superior-nasal segment is the most vulnerable [6, 49, 50].

Different patterns of RNFL and GCC damage reflect different patterns of primary damage to neurons and indicate different mechanisms of vascular disorders in each condition. In GON, changes in the form of arc-shaped defects are consistent with the topography of retinal nerve fibers [51]. In turn, in NAION, the changes are due to the structure of the Zinn-Haller arterial vascular circle, which is formed by the distal branches of the posterior short ciliary arteries and consists of the lower and upper halves [52].

Obviously, the changes in both retinal and choroidal peripapillary blood flow will be different. The decrease in the density of the capillaries of the radial peripapillary plexus in NAION is more pronounced than in GON [53]. A thicker peripapillary choroid is a predisposing factor for the development of NAION [54–56]. Unlike GON, capillary perfusion of the prelaminar tissue induces axonal damage without deformation and damage to lamina cribrosa [57].

Thus, the state of the choroid and lamina cribrosa can be additional differential diagnostic criteria of GON and NAION.

4. Optic neuritis associated with multiple sclerosis

Optic neuritis associated with multiple sclerosis: Multiple sclerosis (MS) is a chronic neurodegenerative disease characterized by demyelination of various parts of the central nervous system caused by (autoimmune) inflammatory processes.

Optic neuritis (ON) is an initial symptom in about 20% of MS patients and occurs in 50% of patients during the course of the disease [58].

The pathological mechanism underlying the decrease in the thickness of RNFL and GC in patients with MS, both with and without previous ON, still remains controversial. However, it is recognized that progressive structural changes are caused by neurodegeneration, not inflammation [59]. There is a correlation between the OCT parameters and the MS manifisattions. RNFL and GCC thinning associated with optical neuropathy in MS correlate not only with visual acuity, and the rate of progression of the disease but also with a lesion of the gray matter of the brain. Therefore, OCT is used to monitor the disease, potentially reducing the need for frequent magnetic resonance imaging [60–64].

The changes in the GCC in MS are ahead of the RNFL changes. Volume and thickness analysis GCC is a more sensitive and reliable indicator of retrobulbar neuroaxonal damage in MS (appears on average after 2 weeks) [3].

The temporal quadrant of the RNFL is more sensitive to damage (**Figure 8**). Lower RNFL values correlate with a decrease in visual acuity, contrast sensitivity, average sensitivity of the visual field, and average indicators of color vision [65].

OCTA demonstrates a decrease in the density of parafoveolar and peripapillary capillaries, respectively, structural damage.

The detection of changes in the paired eye without ON reflects subclinical structural damage of the RNFL. Performing OCT is advisable for monitoring the disease, predicting after relapses of ON, and evaluating the effectiveness of treatment.

Despite the fact that the average thickness of the RNFL and GCC on both sides is within the normative values, the indicators on the right are lower. Local thinning of RNFL (sector 9 h) and GCC by the course of the papillomacular bundle, a decrease in the density of the parafoveolar and peripapillary capillaries along the course of the papillomacular bundle. Diffuse depression of the visual field, central perimetric defect.

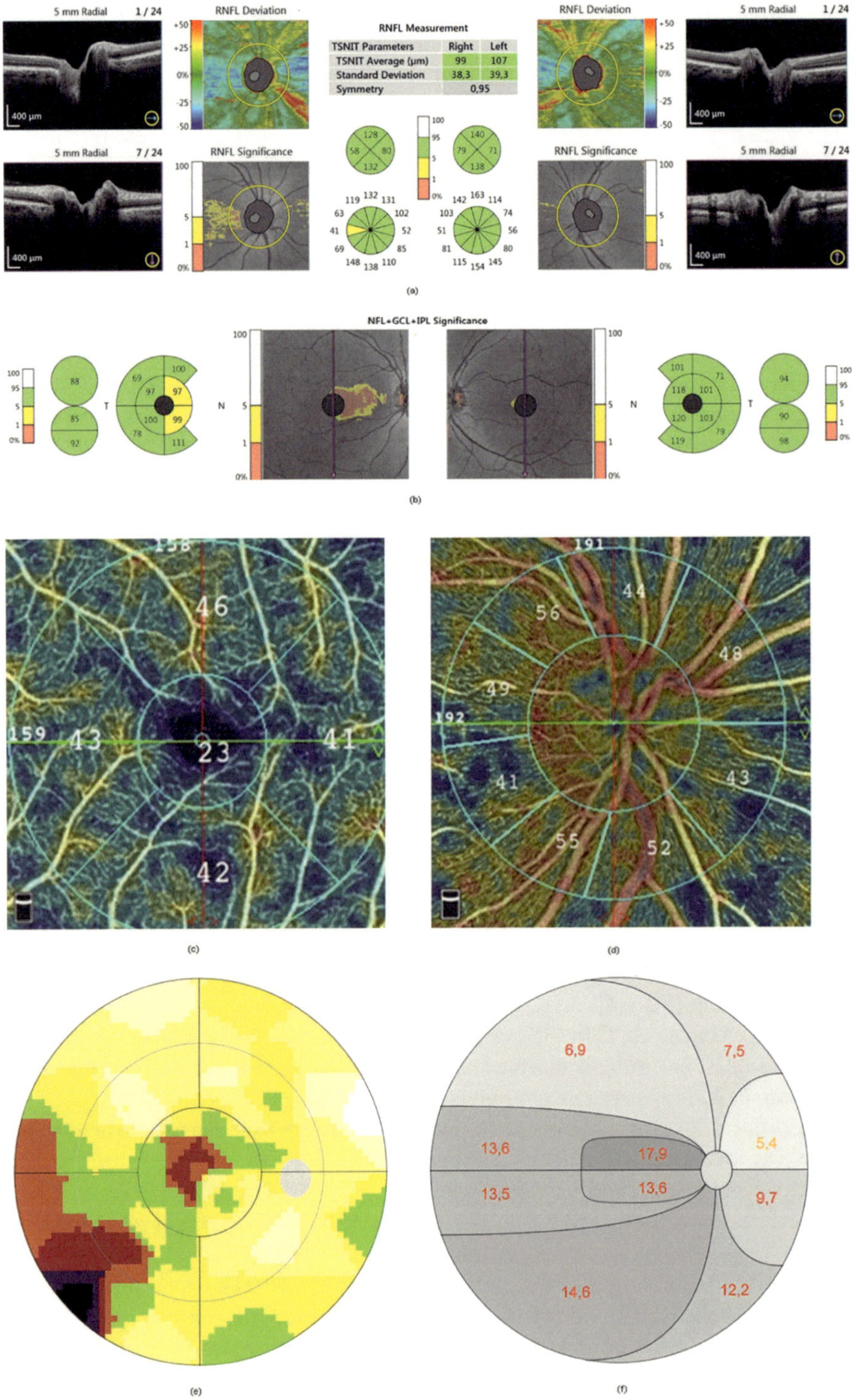

Figure 8.
Man, 42 years old. The MS debut. BCVA 0.5/1.0. A—3D scanning protocol of the OND. B—3D macular scanning protocol. C—OCTA of the superficial plexus and radial peripapillary plexus of the right eye. E—grayscale of values OD. F—cluster analysis OD.

5. Compression optic neuropathy

Compression optic neuropathy (CON) develops more often as a result of compression at the level of the optic nerve (meningioma), orbit (thyroid disease), and anterior segment of the visual pathway (more often at the level of chiasm in pituitary lesions).

If the visual pathway is affected, atrophy can go in the antegrade direction. Experimental studies have proved the existence of retrograde trans-synaptic degeneration of the visual pathway in animals [66, 67].

It was believed that with acquired damage to the central neuron of the human visual pathway, atrophy of the nerve fiber ends at the level of synapses in the external cranial body and does not extend to the anterior segment of the visual pathway [68]. Contrary to this opinion, OCT demonstrates the possibility of the existence of acquired trans-synaptic retrograde degeneration of nerve fibers of the human visual pathway [69, 70]. OCT plays a role not only in the diagnosis and monitoring of compression but also in the prediction of visual functions after surgical treatment.

CON may be detected by OCT earlier than with ophthalmoscopy. A manifestation of the compression effect on the visual tract is the RNFL and GCC thinning. GCC thinning, as a rule, is detected earlier than RNFL changes and standard automated perimeter changes. Hemianopia on perimetry can present as a hemi-macular atrophy on the OCT (**Figure 9**). The excavation increase during compression is due to antegrade degeneration of axons and secondary collapse of glial support tissue [71]. The excavation is usually rounded, central, and not vertically oriented, as in glaucoma (**Figure 10**).

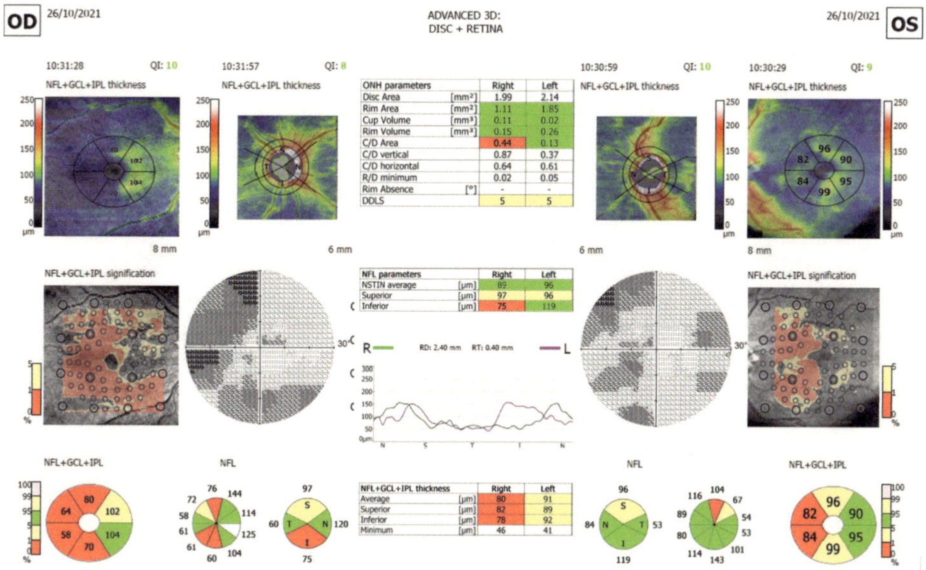

Figure 9.
A 44-year-old woman complained for the first time of a vision reduction in her right eye. BCVA 0.6/1.0. For half of the year, frequent headaches occur. A hemi-muscular atrophy on the OCT, hemianopia on perimetry. Homonymous hemianopia. A neurosurgeon's examination revealed pituitary craniopharyngioma.

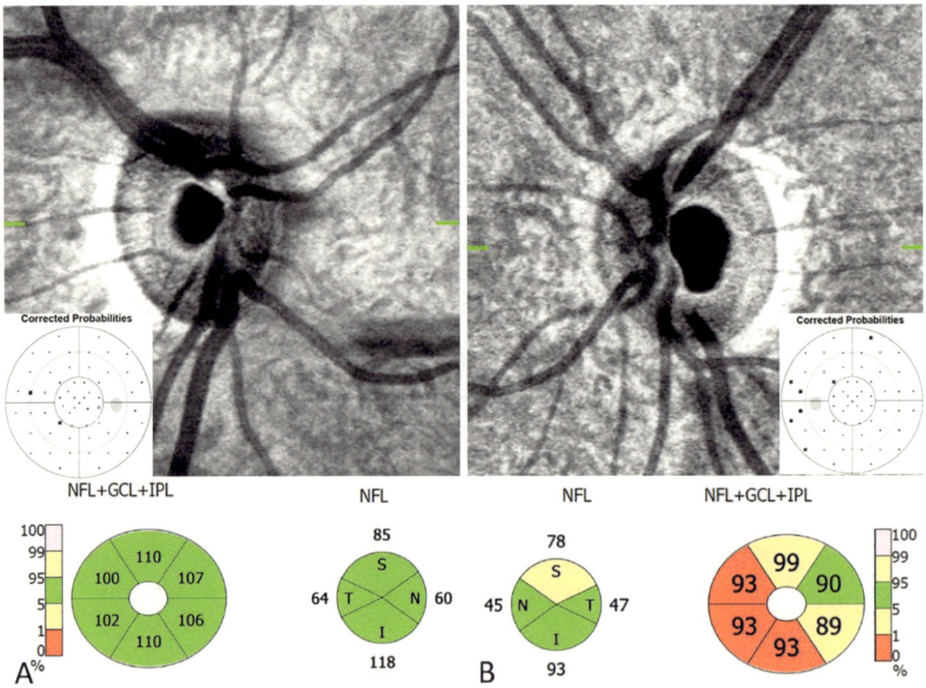

Figure 10.

A 15-year-old girl. Optic nerve glioma of OS (prechiasmal localization, external and internal hydrocephalus. BCVA 1.0/0.9. Increased excavation, RNFL and GCC thinning, and unilateral hemianopsia OS (enface optical disk, perimetry, thickness of SNVS and ganglion complex OD—A and OS—B).

When detecting the asymmetry of the excavation, the RNFL and GCC thickness in symmetrical IOP, OCT may be the key to localizing the compression location [25, 72–79].

Thus, the specific features of CON are decreased visual acuity, vertical defects of the visual field, decoloration of the OND, expansion of excavation, and hemi-macular atrophy on the OCT, age younger than 50 years.

The characteristic pattern of RNFL and GCC damage in optical neuropathies makes it easier to understand the various pathological mechanisms of damage and differentiate early glaucoma changes from other optical neuropathies.

Arcuate inferior temporal defects are a sign of early glaucoma ascending atrophy. Diffuse horizontally oriented loss of RNFL and GCC is a sign of ascending atrophy in NAOIN. Centrally oriented lesions of RNFL, GCC, and visual field defects are formed with descending/ascending atrophy in MS. Homonymous, vertically oriented loss of RNFL and GC is characteristic of descending atrophy in cerebral pathology in the chiasm region.

6. Conclusion

The pattern of changes in RNFL and GCC allows for predicting changes in the visual field and can be used to quantify lesions of the visual pathway in patients with brain dysfunction when it is impossible to perform perimeter tests. The high repeatability and reproducibility of objective retinal biomarkers, and ease of visualization explain the attractiveness and prospects of OCT.

Obviously, OCT is not the only tool for the diagnosis of neurological diseases; however, it can be successfully used in complex diagnostics, often replacing expensive invasive studies. This reduces the burden on patients on the one hand and reduces healthcare costs on the other hand.

Author details

Svetlana Zhukova*, Tatiana Iureva and Dmitry Samsonov
Irkutsk Branch of S.N. Fyoforov "Eye microsurgery" Federal State Institution of Ministry of Health of Russian Federation, Russia

*Address all correspondence to: zhukswetlana@gmail.com

References

[1] Huang JY, Pekmezci M, Mesiwala N, Kao A, Lin S. Diagnostic power of optic disc morphology, peripapillary retinal nerve fiber layer thickness, and macular inner retinal layer thickness in glaucoma diagnosis with fourier-domain optical coherence tomography. Journal of Glaucoma. 2011;**20**:87-95

[2] Park KA, Kim YD, In Woo K, Kee C, Han JC. Optical coherence tomography measurements in compressive optic neuropathy associated with dysthyroid orbitopathy. Graefe's Archive for Clinical and Experimental Ophthalmology. 2016;**254**(8):1617-1624

[3] Kupersmith MJ, Garvin MK, Wang JK, Durbin M, Kardon R. Retinal ganglion cell layer thinning within one month of presentation for optic neuritis. Multiple Sclerosis. 2016;**22**(5):641-648

[4] Fukuchi M, Kishi S, Li D, Akiyama H. Acute ganglion cell loss during rapid visual recovery in optic neuritis. Graefe's Archive for Clinical and Experimental Ophthalmology. 2016;**254**(12):2355-2360

[5] Bock M, Brandt AU, Dörr J, Kraft H, Weinges-Evers N, Gaede G, et al. Patterns of retinal nerve fiber layer loss in multiple sclerosis patients with or without optic neuritis and glaucoma patients. Clinical Neurology and Neurosurgery. 2010;**112**(8):647-652

[6] Lee YH, Kim KN, Heo DW, Kang TS, Lee SB, Kim CS. Difference in patterns of retinal ganglion cell damage between primary open-angle glaucoma and non-arteritic anterior ischaemic optic neuropathy. PLoS One. 2017;**12**(10):e0187093

[7] Fard MA, Afzali M, Abdi P, Yasseri M, Ebrahimi KB, Moghimi S. Comparison of the pattern of macular ganglion cell-inner plexiform layer defect between ischemic optic neuropathy and open-angle glaucoma. Investigative Ophthalmology & Visual Science. 2016;**57**(3):1011-1016

[8] Balk LJ, Twisk JWR, Steenwijk MD, et al. A dam for retrograde axonal degeneration in multiple sclerosis? Journal of Neurology, Neurosurgery, and Psychiatry. 2014;**85**(7):782-789

[9] Smith AM, Czyz CN. Neuroanatomy, cranial nerve 2 (Optic). In: StatPearls [Internet]. Treasure Istland (FL): StatPearls Publishing; Jan 2022. 7 Nov 2022. PMID: 29939684

[10] Lawlor M, Danesh-Meyer H, Levin LA, Davagnanam I, De Vita E, Plant GT. Glaucoma and the brain: Trans-synaptic degeneration, structural change, and implications for neuroprotection. Survey of Ophthalmology. 2018;**63**(3):296-306. DOI: 10.1016/j.survophthal.2017.09.010

[11] Danesh-Meyer HV, Levin LA. Glaucoma as a neurodegenerative disease. Journal of Neuro-Ophthalmology. 2015:35, S22-SS8

[12] Forrester JV, Dick AD, McMenamin PG, Roberts F, Pearlman E. The Eye: Basic Sciences in Practice. 4th ed. London: WB Saunders Ltd.; 2015. p. 568

[13] Weinreb RN, Khaw PT. Primary open-angle glaucoma. Lancet. 2004;**363**(9422):1711-1720. DOI: 10.1016/S0140-6736(04)16257-0

[14] Weinreb RN, Aung T, Medeiros FA. The pathophysiology and treatment of glaucoma: A review. Journal of

the American Medical Association. 2014;**311**(18):1901-1911. DOI: 10.1001/jama.2014.3192

[15] Keltner JL, Johnson CA, Anderson DR, et al. Ocular hypertension treatment study group. The association between glaucomatous visual fields and optic nerve head features in the ocular hypertension treatment study. Ophthalmology. 2006;**113**(9):1603-1612. DOI: 10.1016/j.ophtha.2006.05.061

[16] Medeiros FA, Zangwill LM, Bowd C, Mansouri K, Weinreb RN. The structure and function relationship in glaucoma: Implications for detection of progression and measurement of rates of change. Investigative Ophthalmology & Visual Science. 2012;**53**(11):6939-6946. DOI: 10.1167/iovs.12-10345

[17] Miglior S, Zeyen T, Pfeiffer N, Cunha-Vaz J, Torri V, Adamsons I, et al. Results of the European Glaucoma prevention study. Ophthalmology. 2005;**112**(3):366-375. DOI: 10.1016/j.ophtha.2004.11.030

[18] Medeiros FA, Alencar LM, Zangwill LM, Bowd C, Sample PA, Weinreb RN. Prediction of functional loss in glaucoma from progressive optic disc damage. Archives of Ophthalmology. 2009;**127**(10):1250-1256. DOI: 10.1001/archophthalmol.2009.276

[19] Malik R, Swanson WH, Garway-Heath DF. 'Structure-function relationship' in glaucoma: Past thinking and current concepts. Clinical & Experimental Ophthalmology. 2012;**40**(4):369-380. DOI: 10.1111/j.1442-9071.2012.02770.x

[20] Sánchez-Pulgarín M, Saenz-Frances F, Martinez-de-la-Casa JM, García-Feijoó J, Ferreras-Amez A, Pablo LE. Structure-function relationship in a series of glaucoma cases. Journal Français d'Ophtalmologie. 2020;**43**(2):111-122. DOI: 10.1016/j.jfo.2019.07.009

[21] Vazquez LE, Bye A, Aref AA. Recent developments in the use of optical coherence tomography for glaucoma. Current Opinion in Ophthalmology. 2021;**32**(2):98-104. DOI: 10.1097/ICU.0000000000000733

[22] Tatham AJ, Medeiros FA. Detecting structural progression in glaucoma with optical coherence tomography. Ophthalmology. 2017;**124**(12S):S57-S65. DOI: 10.1016/j.ophtha.2017.07.015

[23] Hood DC, Raza AS, de Moraes CG, Odel JG, Greenstein VC, Liebmann JM, et al. Initial arcuate defects within the central 10 degrees in glaucoma. Investigative Ophthalmology & Visual Science. 2011;**52**(2):940-946. DOI: 10.1167/iovs.10-5803

[24] Hood DC, Raza AS, de Moraes CG, Liebmann JM, Ritch R. Glaucomatous damage of the macula. Progress in Retinal and Eye Research. 2013;**32**:1-21. DOI: 10.1016/j.preteyeres.2012.08.003

[25] Hood DC. Improving our understanding, and detection, of glaucomatous damage: An approach based upon optical coherence tomography (OCT). Progress in Retinal and Eye Research. 2017;**57**:46-75. DOI: 10.1016/j.preteyeres.2016.12.002

[26] Kanamori A, Nakamura M, Tomioka M, Kawaka Y, Yamada Y, Negi A. Structure-function relationship among three types of spectral-domain optical coherent tomography instruments in measuring parapapillary retinal nerve fibre layer thickness. Acta Ophthalmologica. 2013;**91**(3):e196-e202. DOI: 10.1111/aos.12028

[27] Mwanza JC, Budenz DL, Warren JL, Webel AD, Reynolds CE, Barbosa DT, et al. Retinal nerve fibre layer thickness floor and corresponding functional loss in glaucoma. The British Journal of Ophthalmology. 2015;**99**(6):732-737. DOI: 10.1136/bjophthalmol-2014-305745

[28] Ueda K, Kanamori A, Akashi A, Kawaka Y, Yamada Y, Nakamura M. Difference in correspondence between visual field defect and inner macular layer thickness measured using three types of spectral-domain OCT instruments. Japanese Journal of Ophthalmology. 2015;**59**(1):55-64. DOI: 10.1007/s10384-014-0355-z

[29] Kerrigan-Baumrind LA, Quigley HA, Pease ME, Kerrigan DF, Mitchell RS. Number of ganglion cells in glaucoma eyes compared with threshold visual field tests in the same persons. Investigative Ophthalmology & Visual Science. 2000;**41**(3):741-748

[30] Naghizadeh F, Holló G. Detection of early glaucomatous progression with octopus cluster trend analysis. Journal of Glaucoma. 2014;**23**(5):269-275. DOI: 10.1097/IJG.0b013e3182741c69

[31] Mandava S, Zulauf M, Zeyen T, Caprioli J. An evaluation of clusters in the glaucomatous visual field. American Journal of Ophthalmology. 1993;**116**(6):684-691. DOI: 10.1016/s0002-9394(14)73466-x

[32] Lefrançois A, Valtot F, Barrault O. Notre expérience avec le nouveau logiciel d'analyse du champ visuel Octopus Field Analysis (OFA V2.2) [New diagnosis approaches: Our experience with Octopus Field Analysis (OFA V2.2), the new software for analysis of visual field]. Journal of Ophthalmology. 2009;**32**(3):160-171. DOI: 10.1016/j.jfo.2009.03.005

[33] Hood DC, Tsamis E, Bommakanti NK, Joiner DB, Al-Aswad LA, Blumberg DM, et al. Structure-function agreement is better than commonly thought in eyes with early glaucoma. Investigative Ophthalmology & Visual Science. 2019;**60**(13):4241-4248. DOI: 10.1167/iovs.19-27920

[34] Hood DC, De Cuir N, Blumberg DM, Liebmann JM, Jarukasetphon R, Ritch R, et al. A single wide-field OCT protocol can provide compelling information for the diagnosis of early glaucoma. Translational Vision Science & Technology. 2016;**5**(6):4. DOI: 10.1167/tvst.5.6.4

[35] Jia Y, Tan O, Tokayer J, Potsaid B, Wang Y, Liu JJ, et al. Split-spectrum amplitude-decorrelation angiography with optical coherence tomography. Optics Express. 2012;**20**(4):4710-4725. DOI: 10.1364/OE.20.004710

[36] Spaide RF, Fujimoto JG, Waheed NK, Sadda SR, Staurenghi G. Optical coherence tomography angiography. Progress in Retinal and Eye Research. 2018;**64**:1-55. DOI: 10.1016/j.preteyeres.2017.11.003

[37] Yarmohammadi A, Zangwill LM, Diniz-Filho A, Suh MH, Manalastas PI, Fatehee N, et al. Optical coherence tomography angiography vessel density in healthy, glaucoma suspect, and glaucoma eyes. Investigative Ophthalmology & Visual Science. 2016;**57**(9):451-459. DOI: 10.1167/iovs.15-18944

[38] Lin YH, Huang SM, Yeung L, Ku WC, Chen HS, Lai CC, et al. Correlation of visual field with peripapillary vessel density through optical coherence tomography angiography in normal-tension glaucoma. Translational Vision Science & Technology. 2020;**9**(13):26. DOI: 10.1167/tvst.9.13.26

[39] Kong AW, Turner ML, Saifee M, Jethi M, Mora M, Ou Y. A global and sector-based comparison of OCT angiography and visual field defects in glaucoma. Journal of Ophthalmology. 2022;**11**(2022):6182592. DOI: 10.1155/2022/6182592

[40] Zhukova SI, Yureva TN. Pomkina IV/ features of disorders of regional hemodynamics in patients with glaucoma at different levels of intraocular pressure. Practical Medicine. 2018;**3**(114):57-63

[41] Zhukova S. OCT and OCTA: Cases from Clinical Practice. Poland: ARW DK Media Poland Optopol Tecnology. 2020. 188 p. ISBN 978-83-955393-6-7

[42] Hayreh SS. Ischemic optic neuropathy. Progress in Retinal and Eye Research. 2009;**28**(1):34-62. DOI: 10.1016/j.preteyeres.2008.11.002

[43] Tesser RA, Niendorf ER, Levin LA. The morphology of an infarct in nonarteritic anterior ischemic optic neuropathy. Ophthalmology. 2003;**110**(10):2031-2035. DOI: 10.1016/S0161-6420(03)00804-2

[44] Hayreh SS. Anterior ischemic optic neuropathy. Clinical Neuroscience. 1997;**4**(5):251-263

[45] Hamann S, Malmqvist L, Wegener M, Fard MA, Biousse V, et al. Optic disc Drusen studies consortium. Young adults with anterior ischemic optic neuropathy: A multicenter optic disc Drusen study. American Journal of Ophthalmology. 2020;**217**:174-181

[46] Raizada K, Margolin E. Non-arteritic Anterior Ischemic Optic Neuropathy. Treasure Island (FL): StatPearls Publishing; 2022

[47] Bialer OY, Stiebel-Kalish H. Clinical characteristics of progressive nonarteritic anterior ischemic optic neuropathy. International Journal of Ophthalmology. 2021;**14**(4):517-522. DOI: 10.18240/ijo.2021.04.06

[48] Arnold AC, Levin LA. Treatment of ischemic optic neuropathy. Seminars in Ophthalmology. 2002;**17**(1):39-46. DOI: 10.1076/soph.17.1.39.10292

[49] Mastropasqua R, Agnifili L, Borrelli E, Fasanella V, Brescia L, Di Antonio L, et al. Optical coherence tomography angiography of the peripapillary retina in normal-tension glaucoma and chronic nonarteritic anterior ischemic optic neuropathy. Current Eye Research. 2018;**43**(6):778-784. DOI: 10.1080/02713683.2018.1438630

[50] Horowitz J, Fishelzon-Arev T, Rath EZ, Segev E, Geyer O. Comparison of optic nerve head topography findings in eyes with non-arteritic anterior ischemic optic neuropathy and eyes with glaucoma. Graefe's Archive for Clinical and Experimental Ophthalmology. 2010;**248**(6):845-851

[51] Jonas JB, Fernández MC, Stürmer J. Pattern of glaucomatous neuroretinal rim loss. Ophthalmology. 1993;**100**(1):63-68

[52] Olver J, Spalton D, McCartney A. Microvascular study of the retrolaminar optic nerve in man: The possible significance in anterior ischaemic optic neuropathy. Eye. 1990;**4**(1):7-24

[53] Fard MA, Suwan Y, Moghimi S, Geyman LS, Chui TY, Rosen RB, et al. Pattern of peripapillary capillary density loss in ischemic optic neuropathy compared to that in primary open-angle glaucoma. PLoS One. 2018;**13**(1):e0189237. DOI: 10.1371/journal.pone.0189237

[54] Nagia L, Huisingh C, Johnstone J, Kline LB, Clark M, Girard MJ, et al. Peripapillary pachychoroid in

nonarteritic anterior ischemic optic neuropathy. Investigative Ophthalmology & Visual Science. 2016;**57**(11):4679-4685. DOI: 10.1167/iovs.16-19315

[55] Girkin CA. Is nonarteritic ischemic optic neuropathy due to choroidal compression of the prelaminar neurovascular compartment of the optic nerve head? Journal of Neuro-Ophthalmology. 2018;**38**:1-3

[56] Feola AJ, Girkin CA, Ethier CR, Samuels BC. A potential role of acute choroidal expansion in nonarteritic anterior ischemic optic neuropathy. Investigative Ophthalmology & Visual Science. 2022;**63**(4):23. DOI: 10.1167/iovs.63.4.23

[57] Kaur C, Sivakumar V, Foulds WS. Early response of neurons and glial cells to hypoxia in the retina. Investigative Ophthalmology & Visual Science. 2006;**47**(3):1126-1141

[58] Roodhooft JM. Ocular problems in early stages of multiple sclerosis. Bulletin Society Belge Ophtalmology. 2009;**313**:65-68

[59] Fisniku LK, Chard DT, Jackson JS, et al. Gray matter atrophy is related to long-term disability in multiple sclerosis. Annals of Neurology. 2008;**64**(3):247-254

[60] Pillay G, Ganger A, Singh D, Bhatia R, Sharma P, Menon V, et al. Retinal nerve fiber layer and ganglion cell layer changes on optical coherence tomography in early multiple sclerosis and optic neuritis cases. Indian Journal of Ophthalmology. 2018;**66**(1):114-119

[61] Krutzke JF. Rating neurological impairement in multiple sclerosis: Expanded Disability Status Scale (EDSS). Neurology. 1983;**33**:1444-1452

[62] Hemond CC, Bakshi R. Magnetic resonance imaging in multiple sclerosis. Cold Spring Harbor Perspectives in Medicine. 2018;**8**(5):a028969. DOI: 10.1101/cshperspect.a028969

[63] Manogaran P, Hanson JV, Olbert ED, Egger C, Wicki C, Gerth-Kahlert C, et al. Optical coherence tomography and magnetic resonance imaging in multiple sclerosis and neuromyelitis optica spectrum disorder. International Journal of Molecular Sciences. 2016;**17**(11):1894

[64] Lambe J, Saidha S, Bermel RA. Optical coherence tomography and multiple sclerosis: Update on clinical application and role in clinical trials. Multiple Sclerosis Journal. 2019;**2019**:353. DOI: 10.1177/1352458519872751

[65] Walter SD, Ishikawa H, Galetta KM, Sakai RE, Feller DJ, Henderson SB, et al. Ganglion cell loss in relation to visual disability in multiple sclerosis. Ophthalmology. 2012;**119**:1250-1257

[66] Unsold R, Hoyt WF. Band atrophy of the optic nerve: The histology of temporal hemianopsia. Archives of Ophthalmology. 1980;**98**:1637-1638. DOI: 10.1001/archopht.1980.01020040489020 4

[67] Van Buren JM. Trans-synaptic retrograde degeneration in the visual system of primates. Journal of Neurology, Neurosurgery, and Psychiatry. 1963;**26**:402-409. DOI: 10.1136/jnnp.26.5.402

[68] Miller NR. Newman SA transsynaptic degeneration. Archives of Ophthalmology. 1981;**99**(9):1654. DOI: 10.1001/archopht.1981.03930020528032

[69] Jindahra PA, Plant GP. Thinning of the retinal nerve fibre layer in homonymous quadrantanopia: Further

evidence for retrograde trans-synaptic degeneration in the human visual system. Neuroophthalmology. 2012;**36**:79-84. DOI: 10.3109/01658107.2012.674615

[70] Jindahra P, Petrie A. Plant GT the time course of retrograde trans-synaptic degeneration following occipital lobe damage in humans. Brain. 2012;**135**:534-541. DOI: 10.1093/brain/awr324

[71] Portney GL, Roth AM. Optic cupping caused by an intracranial aneurysm. American Journal of Ophthalmology. 1977;**84**(1):98-103

[72] Kanamori A, Nakamura M, Matsui N, Nagai A, Nakanishi Y, Kusuhara S, et al. Optical coherence tomography detects characteristic retinal nerve fiber layer thickness corresponding to band atrophy of the optic discs. Ophthalmology. 2004;**111**:2278-2283. DOI: 10.1016/j.ophtha.2004.05.035

[73] Danesh-Meyer HV, Carroll SC, Foroozan R, Savino PJ, Fan J, Jiang Y, et al. Relationship between retinal nerve fiber layer and visual field sensitivity as measured by optical coherence tomography in chiasmal compression. Investigative Ophthalmology & Visual Science. 2006;**47**:4827-4835. DOI: 10.1167/iovs.06-0327

[74] Costa-Cunha LV, Cunha LP, Malta RF, Monteiro MLR. Comparison of Fourier-domain and time-domain optical coherence tomography in the detection of band atrophy of the optic nerve. American Journal of Ophthalmology. 2009;**147**:56-63.e2. DOI: 10.1016/j.ajo.2008.07.020

[75] Monteiro ML, Cunha LP, Vessani RM. Comparison of retinal nerve fiber layer measurements using stratus OCT fast and regular scan protocols in eyes with band atrophy of the optic nerve and normal controls. Arquivos Brasileiros de Oftalmologia. 2008;**71**:534-539. DOI: 10.1590/S0004-7492008000400013.4

[76] Sun M, Zhang A, Ma C, Chin S, Chen X. Quantitative analysis of retinal layers on three-dimensional spectral-domain optical coherence tomography for pituitary adenoma. PLoS One. 2017;**12**:e0179532. DOI: 10.1371/journal.pone.0179532

[77] Onda E, Cioffi GA, Bacon DR, van Buskirk EM. Microvasculature of the human optic nerve. American Journal of Ophthalmology. 1995;**120**(1):92-102

[78] Lambe J, Murphy OC, Saidha S. Can optical coherence tomography be used to guide treatment decisions in adult or pediatric multiple sclerosis? Current Treat Options in Neurology. 2018;**20**(4):9. DOI: 10.1007/s11940-018-0493-6

[79] Friese MA, Schattling B, Fugger L. Mechanisms of neurodegeneration and axonal dysfunction in multiple sclerosis. Nature Reviews. Neurology. 2014;**10**(4):225-238

Chapter 7

Optic Neuropathies

Amin Zand

Abstract

Optic nerve can be affected by various etiologies of optic neuropathies, and it can appear swollen or pale depending on etiology and duration of the disease. These etiologies are inflammation, ischemia, malignancy, idiopathic intracranial hypertension, toxins, and nutritional deficiency. Peripapillary optical coherence tomography (OCT) is widely performed to detect these diseases and monitor them based on the changes in peripapillary retinal nerve fiber layer (RNFL) thickness. Therefore, nowadays this modality of imaging has become a routine test in follow-up of optic nerve diseases. In this chapter, clinical examinations and main findings of peripapillary OCT in common optic neuropathies are discussed.

Keywords: optic nerve head, optic disc, optic neuropathies, peripapillary, optical coherence tomography, retinal nerve fiber layer

1. Introduction

The new generations of optical coherence tomography (OCT) can reproduce the description of optic disc (including its margin, cup, and rim areas) and makes a quantitative analysis of its surrounding structures, including peripapillary retinal nerve fiber layer (RNFL) thickness in different sectors and quadrants.

OCT is a good diagnostic tool for acquired and congenital optic nerve head diseases. In addition, it can be used for monitoring peripapillary RNFL thickness in some conditions including glaucoma and chronic papilledema. OCT is not only useful in the analysis of the optic nerve disorders but also in some of the central nervous system diseases that impact the optic nerve, too.

About the principles of the optic nerve head OCT, in brief, at first it determines the margin of optic disc automatically, even in patients with peripapillary atrophy. The optic disc size between 1.3–2.5 mm^2 is considered standard, and outside of this range, all measurements represent in gray. Then, the device's software identifies the two most refractive zones of the retina, including the RNFL as the inner boundary and the pigment epithelium as the outer boundary of the peripapillary area, and the thickness of the peripapillary nerve fibers is measured at 3.4 mm from the center of the optic. In optic nerve head OCT printouts, strong reflection of peripapillary layers demonstrates that layers are perpendicular to the light of the imaging device. In contrast, areas with low reflection represent parallel layers with the light (**Figure 1**). The RNFL OCT scan maps represent A-scan data of the RNFL thickness from the center of the optic disc. Furthermore, ganglion cell-inner plexiform layer (GC-IPL) can be scanned, too. In these maps, the RNFL

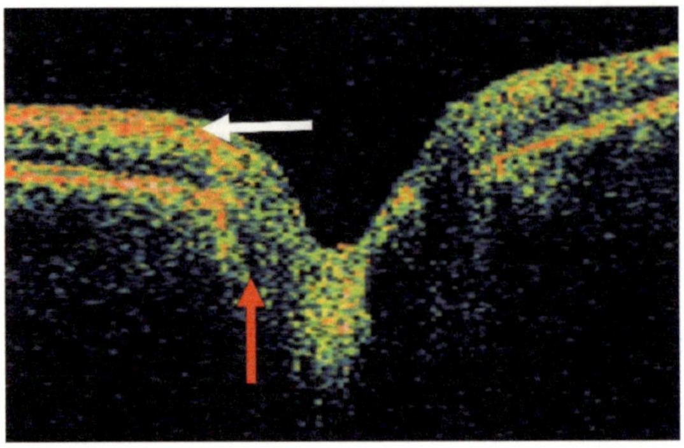

Figure 1.
White arrow: high reflective layers (perpendicular to the light of the OCT device). Red arrow: low reflective layers (parallel to the light).

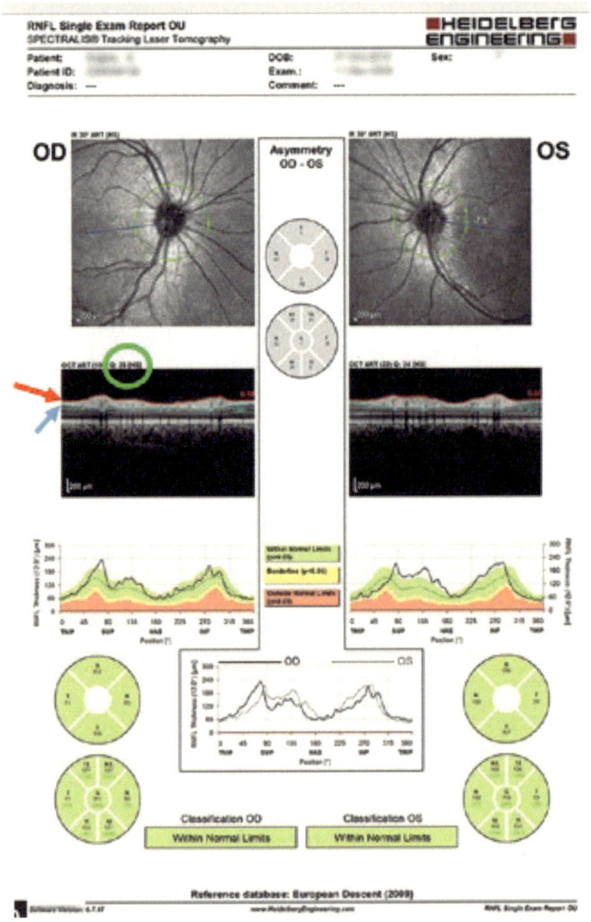

Figure 2.
Peripapillary OCT: green circle: quality score, red arrow: IPL segmentation line, blue arrow: outer boundary of RNFL.

thickness measurements are compared against age-matched normative values. An area where the RNFL thickness is <5% compared to the normal values is shown in yellow and < 1% is shown in red. Before interpretation of the RNFL thickness in these maps, it is necessary to evaluate their accuracy by controlling IPL and RNFL segmentation lines and also quality score of the images (**Figure 2**) [1].

Analysis of the results of optic nerve head OCT needs careful interpretation due to the imaging technique complexity, different aspects of optic nerve head diseases, and potential artifacts. Furthermore, glaucomatous optic neuropathy can mimic neuro-ophthalmology disorders, making challenges in the proper diagnosis.

Some factors may affect the resolution and reliability of optic nerve head OCT images. First, the signal strength (as a quality expresser) of the images must be assessed. For example, it must be >6/10 with the Cirrus™ HD-OCT (Carl Zeiss) device or > 50 with the Optovue (RTVue) device. A poor signal leads to poor quality and misidentification of peripapillary RNFL and their measurements. Second, motion artifacts due to eye movements may cause poor quality, but new devices have programs to resolve this common problem. Third, some ocular conditions may lead to false detection and measurement of peripapillary RNFL. These conditions are including significant cataracts, dense posterior capsular opacity, or increased axial length in pathologic myopia that may influence the measurements [2].

2. Optic neuropathies

2.1 Optic neuritis

Optic neuritis typically occurs in young females, with subacute monocular visual impairment that develops over days. Painful eye movements may present precedes vision impairment. The retrobulbar form (in which the optic disc appears normal) occurs in 2/3 of cases. The most common cause of retrobulbar optic neuritis is multiple sclerosis. In 1/3 of optic neuritis cases, the inflammation involves the anterior portion (papillitis) [3].

During the acute phase of optic neuritis, the RNFL thickness sometimes increased due to mild amounts of edema, which is not clinically detectable. Scatter thinning of the RNFL occurs later until month six after the crisis of the disease (**Figure 3**). In some cases, visual field and OCT parameters may deteriorate and lead to RNFL atrophy [3].

2.2 Papilledema and pseudo papilledema

Optic disc edema describes swelling of the optic nerve head anterior to the lamina cribosa. When disc edema is the result of elevated intracranial pressure, it is labeled papilledema (**Figure 4**).

OCT can be used for differentiating disc edema from pseudo-disc edema. The mean RNFL thickness is significantly greater artificially in patients with true papilledema compared with pseudo papilledema (**Figures 5** and **6**) [4]. But, RNFL assessment by OCT in monitoring optic nerve injury in these patients has some limitations including inaccuracies in detecting true RNFL boundaries in severe cases and identification of coexisting optic atrophy in chronic and long-lasting cases. In these situations ganglion cell complex imaging modality is helpful. This modality of imaging measures the thickness of ganglion cells and inner plexiform layers instead

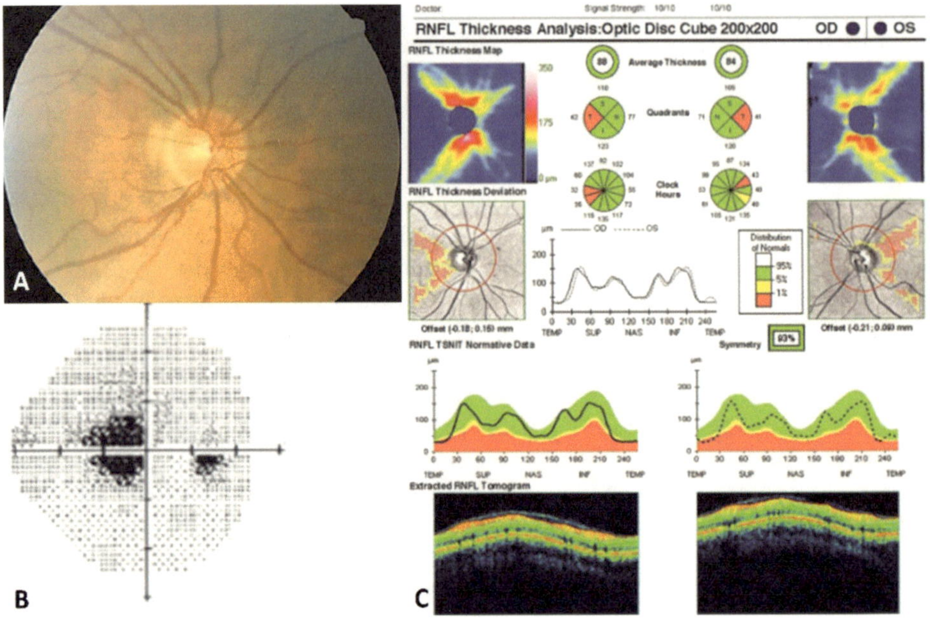

Figure 3.
Retrobulbar optic neuritis: A: optic disc seems to be normal. B: central scotoma is visible. C: OCT shows impairment in the temporal sectors of each eye.

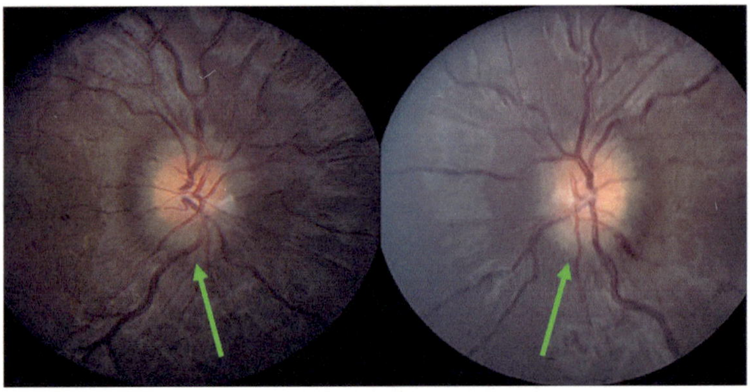

Figure 4.
Swelling of both optic discs (green arrows) in a patient with papilledema.

of just RNFL thickness, which may affect by axonal edema (**Figure 7**) [5]. In OCT angiography (OCTA), dilation and tortuosity of the superficial peripapillary vessels can be detected in acute phases of the disease (**Figure 8**).

One of the causes of pseudo papilledema is optic nerve head drusen (ONHD) which presents with bulblike bodies in the optic nerve head. These bodies may be buried and may consider as true optic disc swelling (**Figure 9**) [6]. In individuals with ONHD, RNFL thickness tends to decrease in quadrants in which drusen are most aggregated (**Figure 10**) [7]. The suggested imaging modalities for differentiating pseudo from true optic disc swelling are optic nerve head B-scan ultrasonography, fluorescein angiography (FA), and OCT [8–11]. In patients with ONHD, ocular B-scan ultrasonography with low gains can detect hyperechoic bodies in the optic

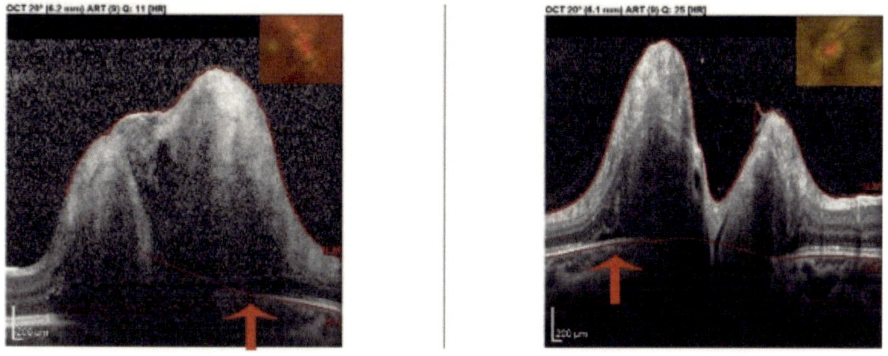

Figure 5.
OCT B-scan of acute papilledema: increased peripapillary thickness with Bruch membrane sloping inward toward the vitreous space of the both eyes (red arrows).

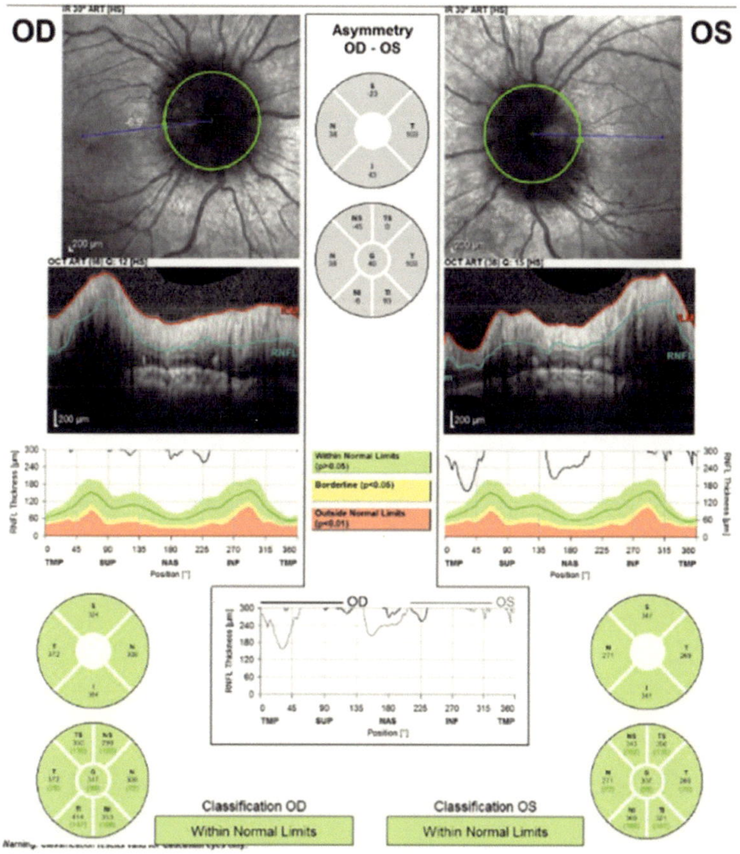

Figure 6.
OCT of acute papilledema: increased RNFL thickness (right eye more than the left): The RNFL edema of the right eye is caused off-the-chart pattern.

nerve head [8]. In autofluorescence, hyperreflective foci can be detectable on the disc. Furthermore, in FA of cases with ONHD just staining of the bodies without leakage is the most common finding, in contrast to the conditions with true optic disc swelling

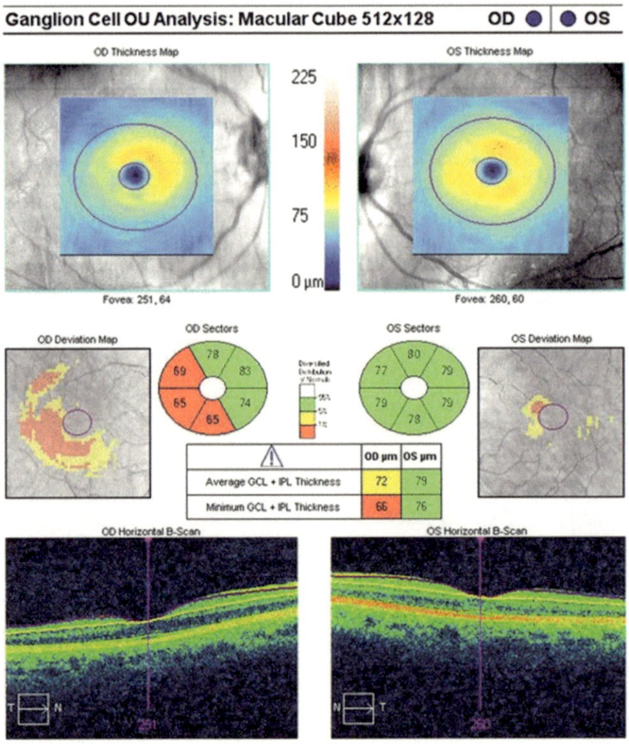

Figure 7.
GCC imaging, 3 months after acute papilledema: the imaging shows a decrease in GCL and IPL layers at temporal and inferior sectors of the right eye.

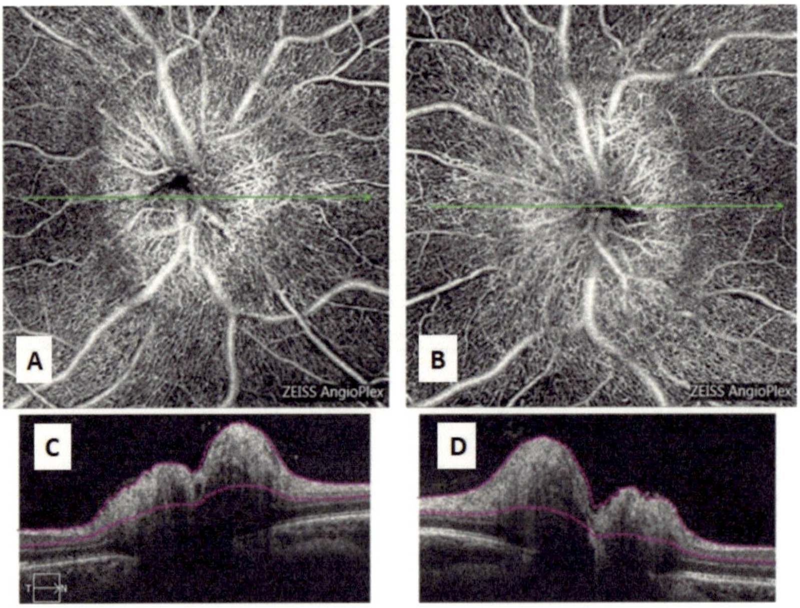

Figure 8.
OCTA of acute papilledema: A and B, Superficial OCTA of both eyes reveal dilation and tortuosity of the superficial peripapillary vessels. C and D, OCT-B scans shows both optic disc elevation.

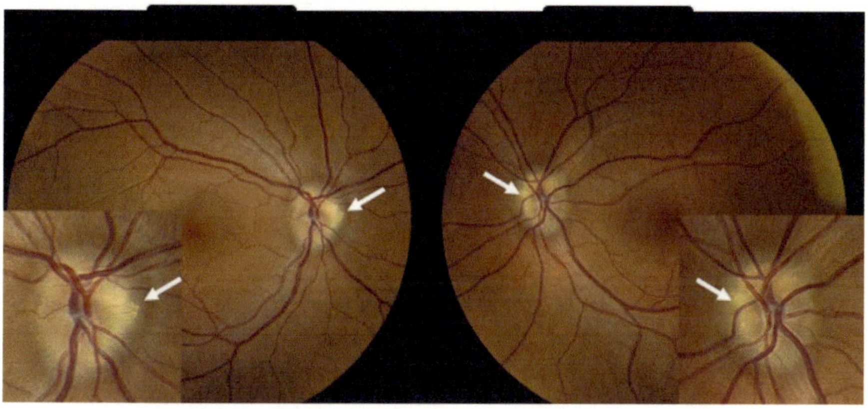

Figure 9.
Bilateral optic nerve head drusen: "lumpy bumpy" appearance of both optic discs with refractile bodies in the disc margins (white arrows).

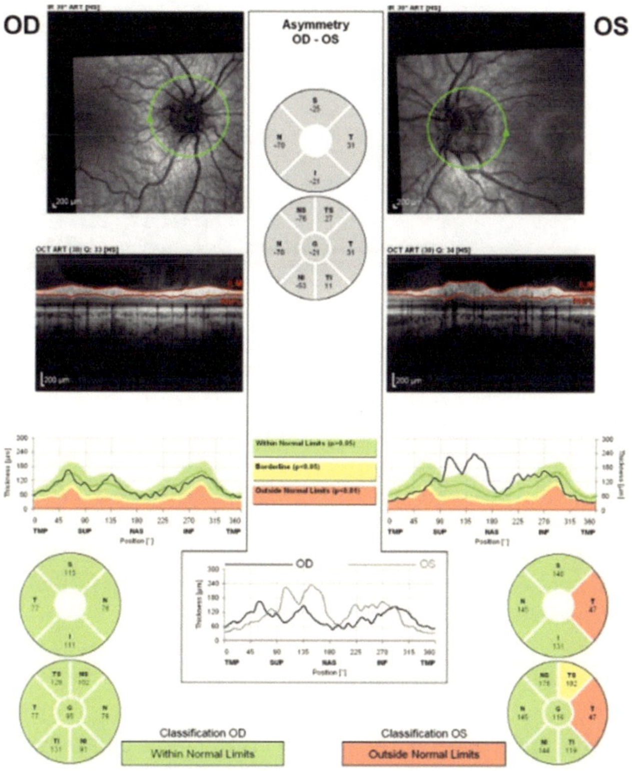

Figure 10.
OCT of bilateral ONHD: Normal RNFL thickness in the right eye with a decrease in temporal RNFL sector of the left eye.

that leakage is common [10–12]. In OCT, most drusens are detected as hypo or hyperreflective signal masses surrounded by hyper-reflective margins. By using OCT, more information about depth of the drusen, its morphology, and its association with surrounding structures can be obtained. In addition, small buried deep drusens

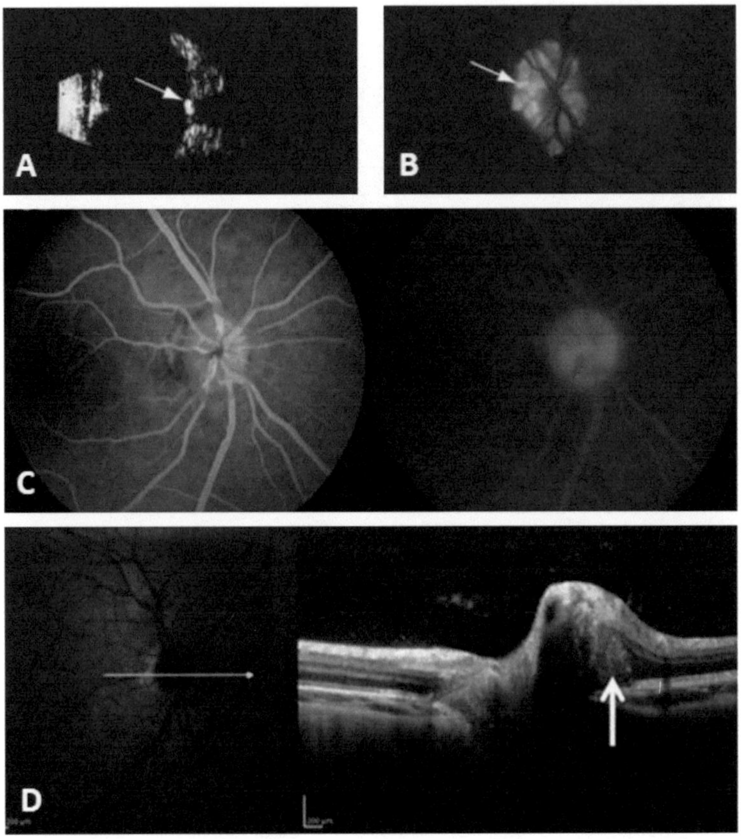

Figure 11.
Optic disc drusen: A, B-scan ultrasonogram, reveal a focal high reflective (due to calcification) elevation within the optic disc (arrow), which persists when the gain is decreased. B, hyper autofluorescence of the drusens are shown (arrow). C, in FA, staining of the drusens without leakage in late phase is detected. D, OCT shows a focal hyper reflective mass (white arrow) with nasal elevation of the optic disc.

can be detected by OCT (**Figure 11**) [13]. OCTA is a noninvasive imaging modality that could be useful in differentiating challenging cases of optic disc edema [14–18]. Previous studies showed in eyes with true axonal swelling due to papilledema, some vessel density values may differ from eyes with pseudo papilledema, but these changes are not consistent [16].

2.3 Anterior ischemic optic neuropathy

Anterior ischemic optic neuropathy (AION) is the most common acute optic neuropathy in patients more than 50 years of age. Patients experience painless monocular vision loss that develops over hours to days. AION is classified as either arteritic (AAION), in which case it is associated with vasculitis, most commonly giant cell arteritis (GCA), or nonarteritic (NAION) [19].

In fundus examination of affected eye, optic disc swelling with peripapillary hemorrhage can be detected. In AAION type, the optic disc seems more pallor in comparison to the NAION type (**Figure 12**). In acute phase of the disease, peripapillary OCT will be showed diffuse edema of RNFL. In chronic phases, the disc and peripapillary area will be atrophic with pale disc and decreased RNFL thickness in OCT of optic

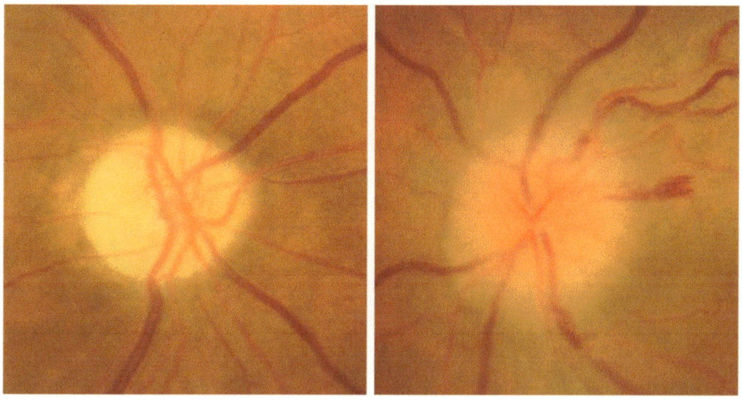

Figure 12.
AION: fundus photography showing atrophy of the right optic disc (old AION) and hyperemic swelling of the left optic disc, with a splinter hemorrhage (acute AION).

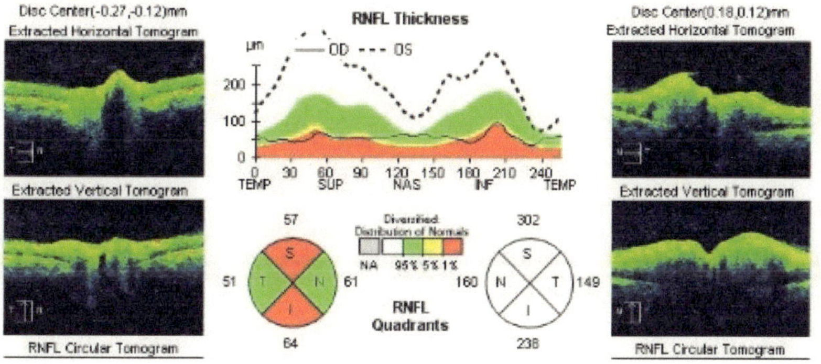

Figure 13.
Peripapillary OCT shows decrease in RNFL thickness at superior and inferior sectors of the right eye (old AION), with diffuse peripapillary RNFL edema of the left eye (acute AION).

nerve head (**Figure 13**) [20]. In FA leakage from the disc can be detected in late phases (**Figure 14**). Although RNFL thickness may increase in both acute NAION and papilledema, by using OCTA these conditions may differ from each other. In eyes with acute NAION due to ischemic condition, some vessel density parameters may decrease, in contrast to conditions without ischemia including acute papilledema (**Figure 15**) [21].

2.4 Infiltrative optic neuropathy

The optic nerve can become infiltrated by primary or secondary tumors and inflammatory processes. Metastases can reach the optic nerve by these routes:

1. from the choroid.

2. by vascular dissemination.

3. by invasion from the orbit.

4. from the central nervous system.

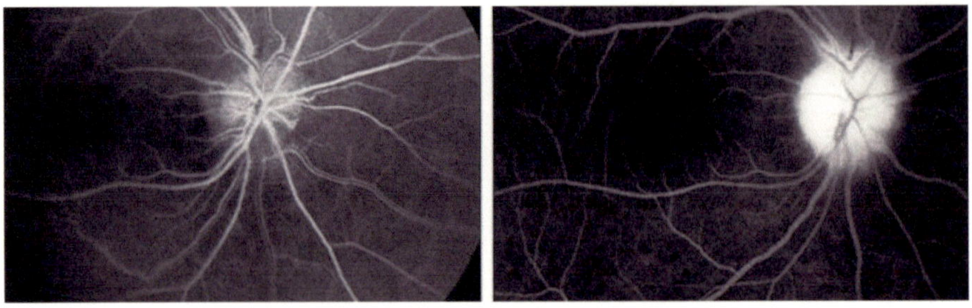

Figure 14.
Acute AION: FA of the right eye shows leakage from the disc in late phase with choroidal filling delay at the nasal side.

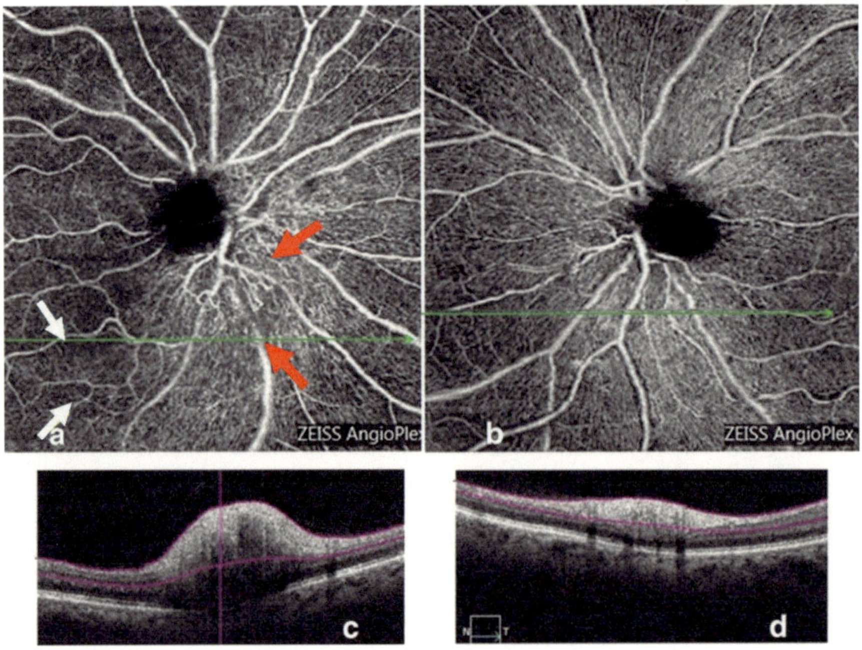

Figure 15.
Acute AION of right eye: a, superficial OCTA right eye demonstrates dilation and tortuosity of the nasal capillaries (red arrows). On the temporal side, dark areas compatible with capillary drop out (white arrow). c, the B-scan OCT shows the disc elevation. In the fellow eye (b and d), the peripapillary capillaries seems to be normal with normal contour of the disc.

The most common metastatic tumors to the optic nerve are adenocarcinomas:

- In females, breast and lung cancers are the most common causes.
- In males, carcinomas of the lung and intestinal tract are the most common causes.
- When the metastasis is located in the orbital portion of the optic nerve:
- The optic disc is usually swollen.

- A yellow-white infiltrative mass can be seen on the optic disc that protruded from the surface of the nerve (**Figure 16**).

- Sometimes tumor cells can be seen in the vitreous body.

B-Scan ultrasonography can reveal abnormal increase in the optic nerve sheath diameter. In peripapillary OCT, an increase in RNFL thickness can be detected. FA of the affected eye may detect a hyperfluorescent mass on the optic disc with no sign of leakage (**Figure 17**) [22, 23].

2.5 Toxic optic neuropathy

Toxic optic neuropathies typically present with a gradually progressive, bilaterally symmetric, painless vision loss affecting central vision. Poisoning with heavy

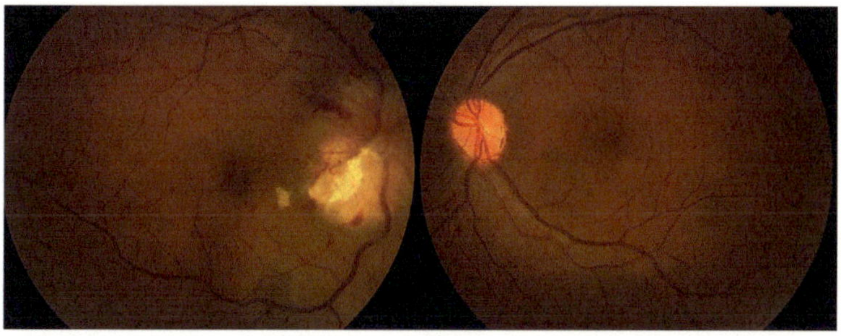

Figure 16.
Infiltrative optic neuropathy: fundus photography of both eyes. The right eye, optic disc swelling with obscuration of blood vessels and prepapillary flamed shape hemorrhage. A large yellowish infiltrative mass, with disruption of the architecture of the optic disc is seen on that. The left eye seems to be normal.

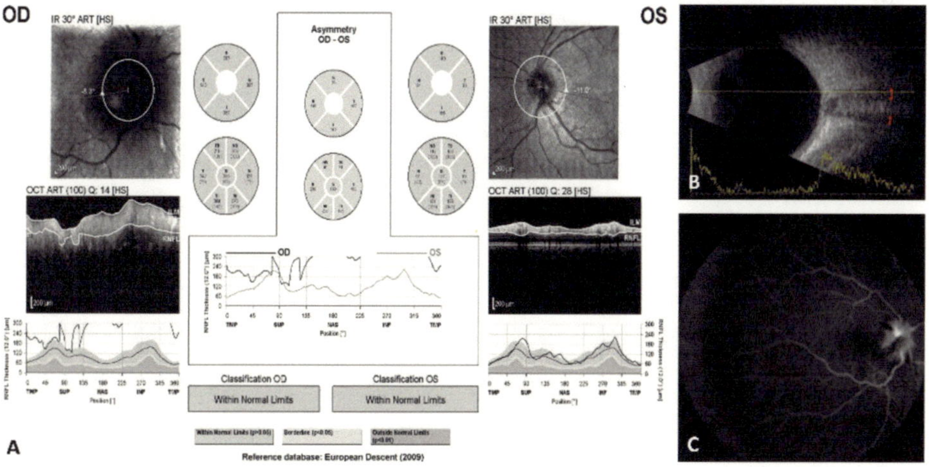

Figure 17.
Infiltrative optic neuropathy: A, peripapillary OCT of both eye. The right eye, increased thickness of RNFL in all four quadrants. The left eye, normal RNFL thicknesses in all sectors. B, B-scan ultrasonography of the right eye reveals abnormally increased optic nerve sheath diameter (red double-headed arrows). C, in FA a hyperfluorescent mass on the right optic disc with no evidence of leakage is visible.

metals like lead can cause toxic optic neuropathy. Patients can be presented with bilateral optic disc swelling and peripapillary hemorrhage, which can be confirmed in peripapillary OCT imaging (**Figures 18** and **19**). In visual field analysis, patients may

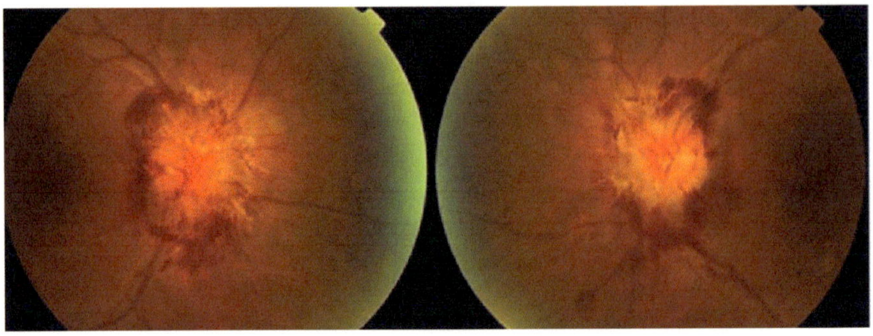

Figure 18.
Acute toxic optic neuropathy in a patient with lead poisoning: fundus photographs show significant hyperemia and edema of both optic discs.

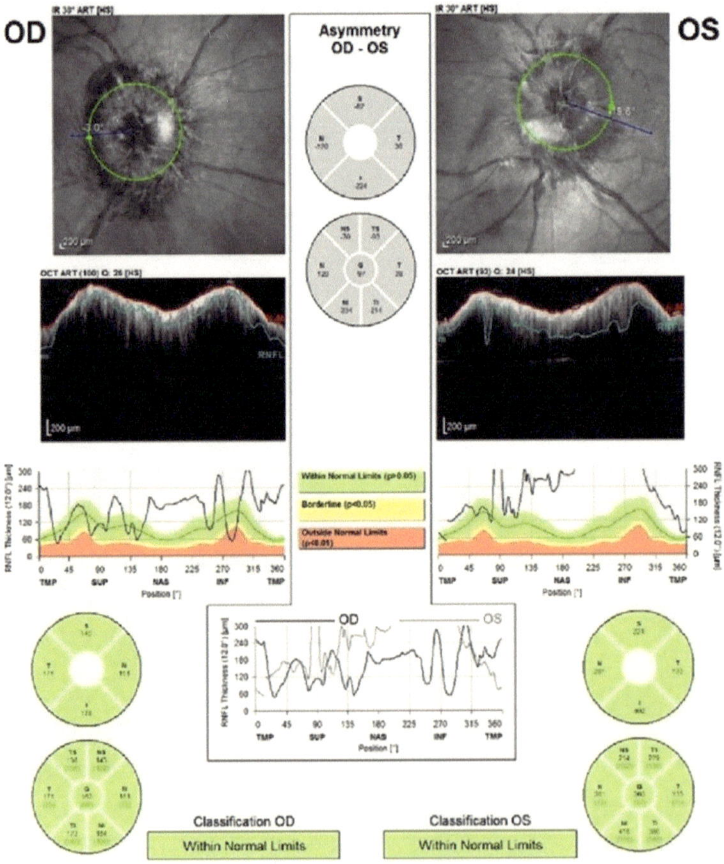

Figure 19.
Peripapillary OCT of a patient with lead poisoning: increased RNFL thickness in all sectors in both eyes is visible, suggestive of bilateral disc edema.

have cecocentral or central scotomas. In FA leakage from the optic nerve head can be detected (**Figure 20**) [24].

2.6 Leber hereditary optic neuropathy

Leber hereditary optic neuropathy (LHON) is the most common inherited mitochondrial disorder and typically affects young males. It typically begins as a unilateral progressive optic neuropathy with sequential involvement of the fellow eye months to years later. Fundus examination may initially reveal normal or pseudo-edematous optic nerves and telangiectatic peripapillary vessels (**Figure 21**) [25]. In late phases, the affected optic disc becomes pale and atrophic. Peripapillary OCT shows axonal swelling, which occurs during the acute phase of the disease (**Figure 22**). Furthermore, OCT clearly detects atrophy of the RNFL following the acute event [26]. In some asymptomatic eyes, OCT may demonstrate an increased RNFL thickness of the temporal quadrant (papillo-macular bundle). In FA of acute involved optic nerve head, no leakage is detected. OCTA may reveal peripapillary telangiectasia in acute phase, followed by capillary dropout, especially in the papillo-macular bundle and also disc cupping (**Figure 23**) [27].

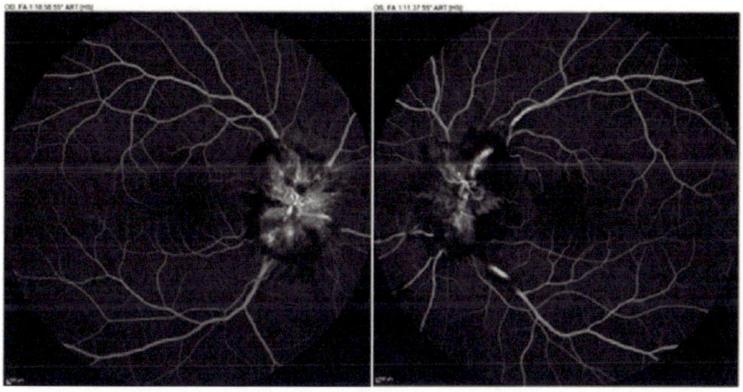

Figure 20.
FA of the same patient with lead poisoning: both discs have leakage, suggestive of bilateral disc swelling.

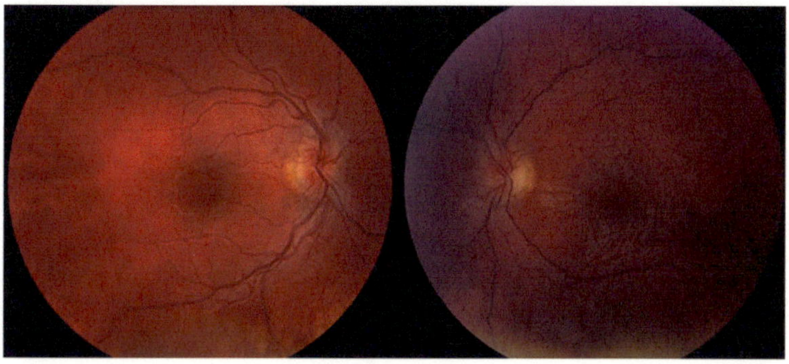

Figure 21.
LHON: right optic disc seems to be elevated with peripapillary telangiectatic vessels. About the left optic disc, it has mild temporal pallor.

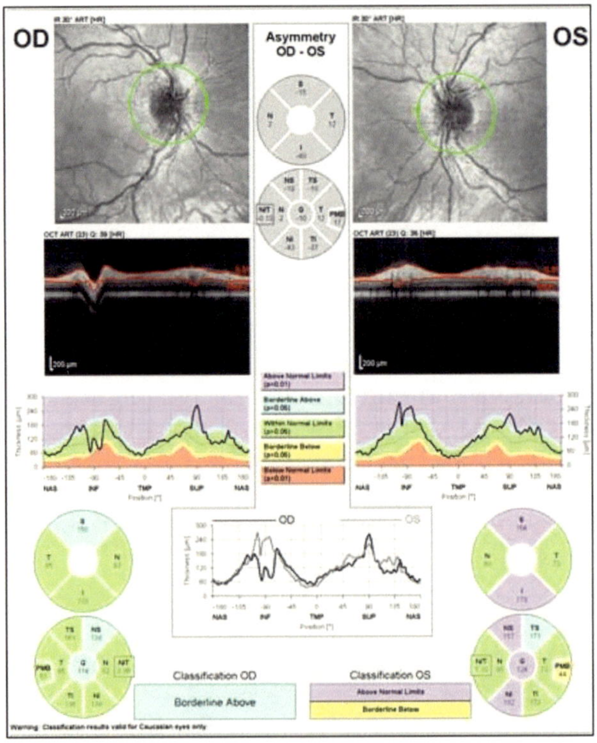

Figure 22.
OCT of LHON: mild peripapillary sectoral RNFL edema in both eyes with a decrease in temporal sector of peripapillary RNFL thickness in the left eye.

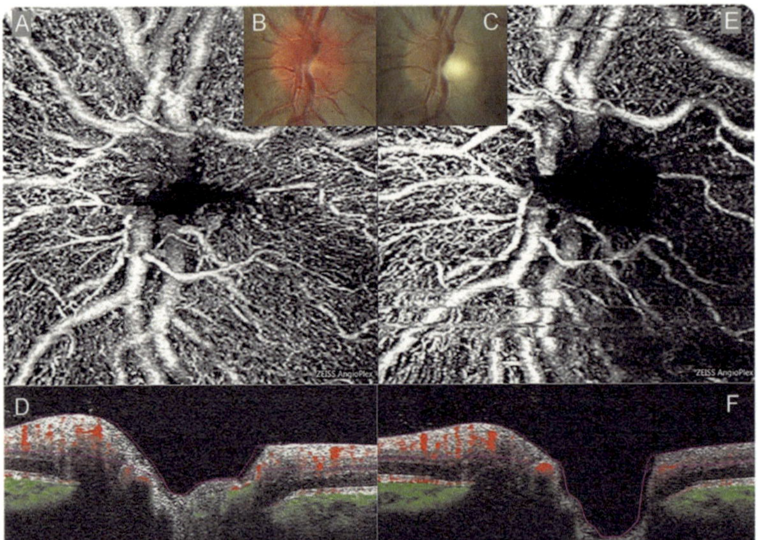

Figure 23.
OCTA of LHON: A, B, C, acute phase of the disease. Optic disc is hyperemic with peripapillary telangiectatic vessels. C, E, F, three months after the onset of the signs, significant capillary dropouts in the temporal side (papillo-macular bundle) and disc cupping are visible.

2.7 Optic pit

Optic pit is a kind of excavated optic disc anomaly. An optic pit is a depression of the optic disc surface that is often gray or white. It is located infero-temporally, and associated with a mild visual field defect (usually paracentral or arcuate) (**Figure 24**). A reduction in RNFL thickness in the excavated sector of the affected optic disc can be seen in peripapillary OCT (**Figure 25**). Serous detachment of the macula develops in 25–75% of optic pit cases, possibly related to liquefied vitreous entering the sub-retinal space through communication between the optic pit and the macula [28, 29].

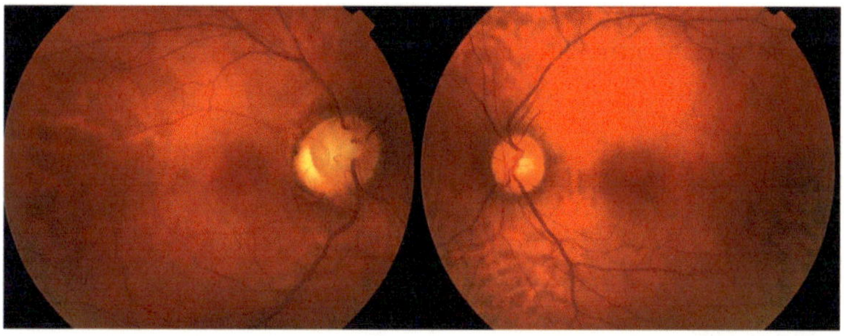

Figure 24.
Fundus photography of both eyes: a yellow-whitish excavation at the inferotemporal rim of the optic disc of right eye. The left optic disc seems to be normal.

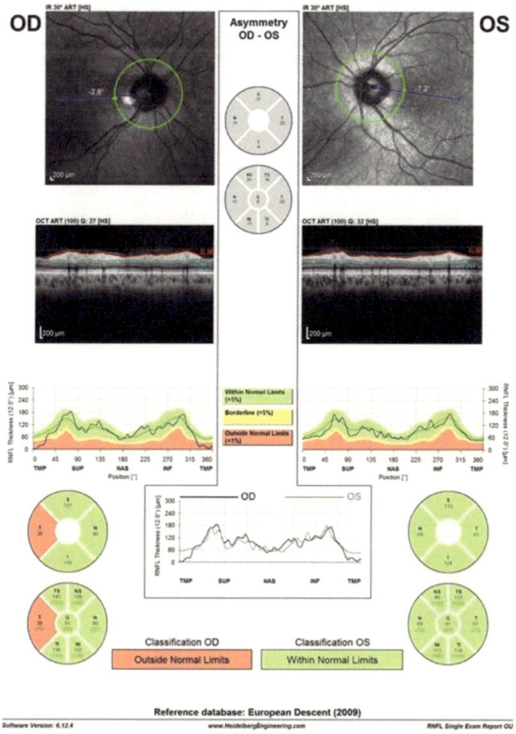

Figure 25.
A significant reduction in RNFL thickness in the temporal sector of right eye is visible. Coloboma is clearly seen on vertical OCT scan as well as horizontal scans through right optic pit.

3. Conclusion

By optic nerve head OCT, different structures are being studied and measured. This imaging modality can analyze not only layers' thickness but also their contents.

Peripapillary OCT is widely used to detect optic neuropathies. Changes in peripapillary RNFL thickness are important in serial OCTs. This modality of imaging is available and enough reliable in diagnosis of optic nerve head diseases in routine clinical practice.

Although optic nerve head OCT is developing constantly, we cannot replace it with other tests including visual field analysis, especially in glaucoma patients.

A combination of OCT and OCTA findings will allow an understanding of complex pathologies involving the optic nerve head and peripapillary areas.

Acknowledgements

I thank Dr. Kaveh Abri Aghdam for sharing the images.

Conflict of interest

The author has no conflict of interest to declare.

Author details

Amin Zand
Department of Ophthalmology, Shafa Hospital, Kerman University of Medical Sciences, Kerman, Iran

*Address all correspondence to: sandpost3@gmail.com

References

[1] La Bruna S, Rai A, Mao G, et al. The OCT RNFL probability map and artifacts resembling glaucomatous damage. Translational Vision Science & Technology. 2022;**11**:18

[2] Nordmann J-P. OCT and Optic Nerve. First. Paris, France: Laboratoire Théa; 2013

[3] Lamirel C, Newman NJ, Biousse V. Optical coherence tomography (OCT) in optic neuritis and multiple sclerosis. Revue Neurologique (Paris). 2010;**166**:978-986

[4] Heidary G, Rizzo JF. Use of optical coherence tomography to evaluate papilledema and Pseudopapilledema. Seminars in Ophthalmology. 2010;**25**:198-205

[5] Athappilly G, García-Basterra I, Machado-Miller F, et al. Ganglion cell complex analysis as a potential indicator of early neuronal loss in idiopathic intracranial hypertension. Neuro-Ophthalmology. 2019;**43**:10-17

[6] Palmer E, Gale J, Crowston JG, et al. Optic nerve head Drusen: An update. Neuro-Ophthalmology. 2018;**42**:367-384

[7] Bassi S, Mohana K. Optical coherence tomography in papilledema and pseudopapilledema with and without optic nerve head drusen. Indian Journal of Ophthalmology. 2014;**62**:1146

[8] Tuğcu B, Özdemir H. Imaging methods in the diagnosis of optic disc Drusen. Türk Oftalmol Derg. 2016;**46**:232-236

[9] Johnson LN. Differentiating optic disc edema from optic nerve head Drusen on optical coherence tomography. Archives of Ophthalmology. 2009;**127**:45

[10] Chang MY, Velez FG, Demer JL, et al. Accuracy of diagnostic imaging modalities for classifying pediatric eyes as papilledema versus Pseudopapilledema. Ophthalmology. 2017;**124**:1839-1848

[11] Pineles SL, Arnold AC. Fluorescein angiographic identification of optic disc Drusen with and without optic disc edema. J Neuro-Ophthalmology. 2012;**32**:17-22

[12] Cartlidge NE, Ng RC, Tilley PJ. Dilemma of the swollen optic disc: A fluorescein retinal angiography study. The British Journal of Ophthalmology. 1977;**61**:385-389

[13] Guo X, Wu Y, Wu Y, et al. Detection of superficial and buried optic disc drusen with swept-source optical coherence tomography. BMC Ophthalmology. 2022;**22**:219

[14] Akil H, Falavarjani K, Sadda S, et al. Optical coherence tomography angiography of the optic disc; an overview. J. Ophthalmic Vis. Res. 2017;**12**:98

[15] Fard MA, Jalili J, Sahraiyan A, et al. Optical coherence tomography angiography in optic disc swelling. American Journal of Ophthalmology. 2018;**191**:116-123

[16] Fard MA, Sahraiyan A, Jalili J, et al. Optical coherence tomography angiography in papilledema compared with Pseudopapilledema. Investig Opthalmology Vis Sci. 2019;**60**:168

[17] Abri Aghdam K, Ashraf Khorasani M, Soltan Sanjari M, et al. Optical coherence tomography angiography features of optic nerve head

drusen and nonarteritic anterior ischemic optic neuropathy. Canadian Journal of Ophthalmology. 2019;**54**:495-500

[18] Anvari P, Sardarinia M, Zand A, et al. Accuracy of peripapillary OCTA in patients with acute nonarteritic anterior ischemic optic neuropathy. Canadian Journal of Ophthalmology. Epub ahead of print. 2022;**e190-e199**:1-5

[19] Hayreh SS. Management of ischemic optic neuropathies. Indian Journal of Ophthalmology. 2011;**59**:123-136

[20] Ho JK, Stanford MP, Shariati MA, et al. Optical coherence tomography study of experimental anterior ischemic optic neuropathy and histologic confirmation. Investig Opthalmology Vis Sci. 2013;**54**:5981

[21] Gandhi U, Chhablani J, Badakere A, et al. Optical coherence tomography angiography in acute unilateral nonarteritic anterior ischemic optic neuropathy: A comparison with the fellow eye and with eyes with papilledema. Indian Journal of Ophthalmology. 2018;**66**:1144

[22] Takkar A, Naheed D, Dogra M, et al. Infiltrative optic neuropathies: Opening doors to sinister pathologies. Neuro-Ophthalmology. 2017;**41**:279-283

[23] Aghdam KA, Zand A, Sanjari MS. Isolated unilateral infiltrative optic neuropathy in a patient with breast cancer. Turkish J Ophthalmol. 2019;**49**:171-174

[24] Abri Aghdam K, Zand A, Soltan SM. Bilateral optic disc edema in a patient with Lead poisoning. J. Ophthalmic Vis. Res. 2019;**14**:513-517

[25] Lam BL. Leber hereditary optic neuropathy gene therapy clinical trial recruitment. Archives of Ophthalmology. 2010;**128**:1129

[26] Hedges TR, Gobuty M, Manfready RA, et al. The optical coherence tomographic profile of Leber hereditary optic neuropathy. Neuroophthalmology. 2016;**40**:107-112

[27] De Rojas JO, Rasool N, Chen RWS, et al. Optical coherence tomography angiography in Leber hereditary optic neuropathy. Neurology. 2016;**87**:2065-2066

[28] Ohno-Matsui K, Hirakata A, Inoue M, et al. Evaluation of congenital optic disc pits and optic disc Colobomas by swept-source optical coherence tomography. Investig Opthalmology Vis Sci. 2013;**54**:7769

[29] Michalewski J, Michalewska Z, Nawrocki J. Spectral domain optical coherence tomography morphology in optic disc pit associated maculopathy. Indian Journal of Ophthalmology. 2014;**62**:777-781

Chapter 8

Optical Coherence Tomography Angiography (OCT-A): Emerging Landscapes in Neuro-Ophthalmology and Central Nervous System (CNS) Disorders

Mobin Ibne Mokbul

Abstract

Optical Coherence Tomography (OCT) is now being widely used in several branches of biomedical science ranging from ophthalmology to neurology. Emerging from it, optical coherence tomography angiography (OCT-A) is a noninvasive, depth-resolved imaging tool for the visualization of retinal vascular changes. In the field of neuro-ophthalmology, OCT-A proves to be superior than the conventional Fluorescein angiography (FA) or indocyanine green angiography (ICGA). This chapter discussed the role of OCT-A in different neuro-ophthalmological and central nervous system (CNS) disorders including multiple sclerosis, non-arteritic anterior ischemic optic neuropathy (NAION), papilledema, papillitis, glaucoma, Parkinson's disease, Alzheimer's disease, cerebral small vessel diseases, and stroke. Since neuro-ophthalmological and some neurologic conditions show consistent peripapillary and macular capillary changes, OCT-A can be a future useful tool in a physician's armamentarium due to its capability for better delineation of the superficial and deeper retinal and choroidal vasculatures. Furthermore, its limitations, technical challenges, and future research directions are illustrated in this chapter.

Keywords: OCT-A, neurology, neuro-ophthalmology, angiography, optical coherence tomography, Parkinson, stroke, Alzheimer's, multiple sclerosis, neuromyelitis optica, optic nerve, papilledema

1. Introduction

Recent advances in biomedical imaging have led several imaging modalities to improve our understanding of various ophthalmological and/or neurological diseases. First developed by Fujimoto's group at the Massachusetts Institute of Technology (MIT) in 1991, Optical Coherence Tomography (OCT) works based on tissue backscattering properties [1]. OCT utilizes the short coherence length of broad-spectrum light sources to obtain cross-sectional images of biological tissue samples on a microscopic scale. Since its inception in the 1990s, it has rapidly become a crucial imaging technique in various biomedical fields, particularly in ophthalmology, where it can be used to visualize the anterior eye and retina through transparent media. As the brain and retina originate from the same embryologic origin, the retina provides a unique "window" into the central nervous system (CNS) because of having unmyelinated axons and a low concentration of glial cells. That is why retina is called "a relative vacuum" while studying neurons and axons and it can serve as a valuable surrogate marker of neurodegeneration, neuroprotection, and neurorestoration [2].

The major users of OCT technology over the last 20 years have been mostly ophthalmologists, but in these days, it is also being used widely by more specifically neuro-ophthalmologists and neurologists on patients with ocular and/or neurologic disorders. We previously summarized the updates on OCT's applications in neuroscience and interested readers may refer to it [2]. Besides, one of the modern-day OCT successors, OCT Angiography (OCT-A) has drawn significant attention from biomedical communities for its unique capabilities in imaging microvasculature in different neuro-ophthalmological and neurological conditions. Some purely neuro-ophthalmological conditions (e.g., optic neuropathies, papilledema, glaucoma) and some neurologic conditions with ocular manifestations (e.g., multiple sclerosis, Parkinson's disease, Alzheimer's disease, stroke) show changes in eye vasculature that can be detected, studied and monitored using OCT-A, are discussed together in this chapter due to their significant inter-relations [3–9].

In neuro-ophthalmology, OCT-A has been used in different types of optic nerve head (ONH) edema (e.g., ischemic, inflammatory, papilledema) and optic neuropathies (e.g., ischemic, inflammatory, hereditary) [10, 11]. There has been recent attention to implementing OCT-A in diabetic retinopathy as well [12, 13]. The key advantage OCT-A provides in addition to conventional structural OCT images, it can capture the microvascular architecture in unprecedented detail which can synergize the clinical diagnosis, monitoring disease progression and prognosis [14, 15]. Again, some central nervous system (CNS) diseases have retinal microvasculature involvement. For instance, neurodegenerative diseases like Alzheimer's disease (AD) affects retina as well. The mechanism behind the reduced retinal vessel density in AD is not clear, but it has been proposed that decreased angiogenesis due to sequestration of vascular endothelial growth factor (VEGF) by Aβ plaques and competition between Aβ and VEGF receptor 2 is a factor. Studies have found Aβ plaques in the retinas of post-mortem AD patients and in mice with AD. These findings suggest that Optical Coherence Tomography Angiography (OCT-A) could be used to detect microvascular abnormalities in even pre-clinical AD pathology [8]. Recent applications of OCT-A have shed light on acute stroke diagnosis even from retina though it requires further research [7]. In this chapter, we will explore the potential applications of OCT-A in these fields, their challenges, and future directions.

2. Basic concepts of OCT-A

OCT-A is an imaging tool for visualizing the retinal vasculature in the eye based on the traditional OCT but allows for high-speed imaging acquisition of the retinal blood vessels. OCT-A uses algorithms such as Ultrahigh-sensitive optical microangiography, split-spectrum amplitude-decorrelation angiography, full spectrum amplitude decorrelation algorithm, etc. These algorithms produce three-dimensional images of the retinal vasculature in less than 3 seconds. The images are created by taking repeated B-scans of the same cross-section of the eye and detecting changes in the phase and intensity of the OCT signal caused by the movement of red blood cells. OCT-A systems can be used to acquire images with a field of view larger than 6×6 mm, with varying levels of lateral resolution [5]. Images with a wider field of view and improved lateral resolution can be obtained by using a high-speed Swept Source (SS) OCT-A system or wide-field montages (**Figures 1** and **2**).

In addition to traditional OCT functions, OCT-A technology allows for the analysis of multiple retinal layers and corresponding vasculatures, including the inner retina, middle retina, outer retina, choriocapillaris, and choroid. This enables the examination of various vascular features, such as the presence of neovascularization, increased tortuosity, and areas of capillary loss. Quantitative analysis, such as measuring the area of the foveal avascular zone (FAZ) and the relative density, can also be performed using methods like fractal analysis or pixel counting. The flow rate, which is the average decorrelation value of sequential B-scans, can also be used as a surrogate for blood flow rate. The Optovue™ system includes an analysis package that automatically analyzes the FAZ and vessel density in different retinal sub-regions [5]. **Table 1** shows some common OCT-A parameters.

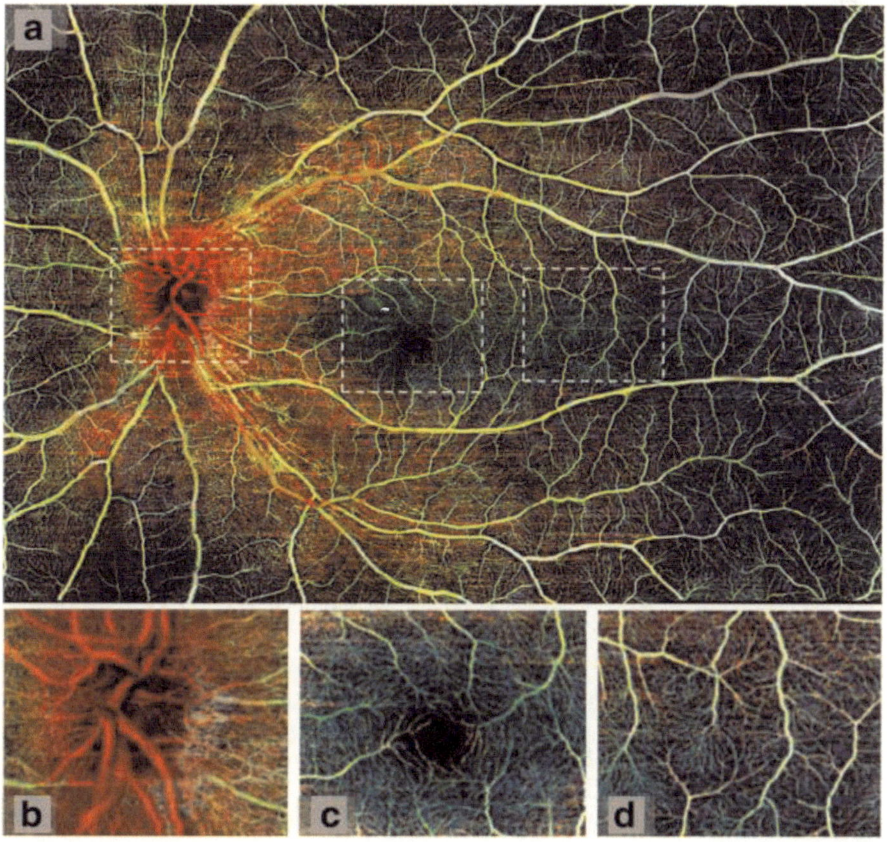

Figure 1.
Wide field montage of healthy retinal microvasculature. The retinal nerve fiber layer is shown in red, the ganglion cell and inner plexiform layers are shown in green, and the inner nuclear and outer plexiform layers are shown in blue. (b), the fovea (c), and (d), the temporal region are all indicated by white boxes. (Reprinted from ref. [14]).

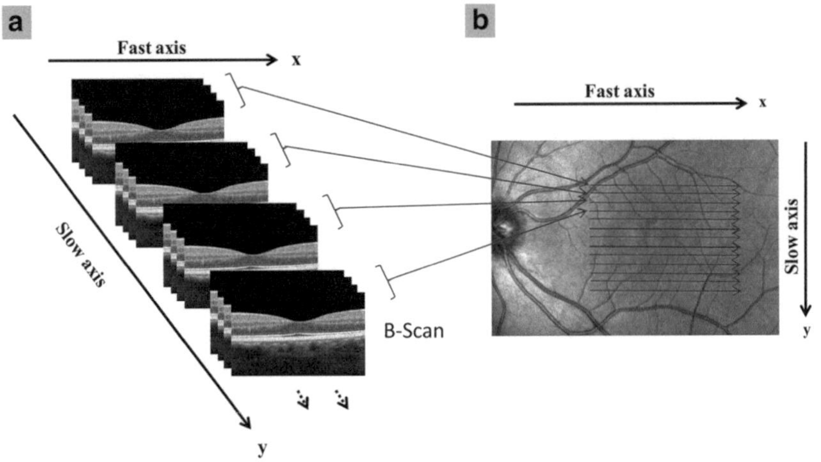

Figure 2.
General scanning protocol for optical coherence tomography angiography (OCT-A). (a) To find the relative flow signal, several B-scans are performed on the "x" fast axis at each of the "y" slow scan axis points. (b) Top view of the same basic scan pattern as in (a), with multiple B-scans performed along each "y" location of the slow axis on the fast axis. AngiovueTM OCT-A was used to obtain sample scans. (a, b). Reprinted from ref. [5].

Parameter	Definition
Vessel length density*	Length-based measurement of vessel density: total length of the perfused vasculature per unit area in the region of measurement (Zeiss definition)
Vessel density*	Area-based measurement of vessel density: expresses how much area is taken up by vessels (Optovue definition)
Perfusion density	Area-based measurement of vessel density: total area of the perfused vasculature per unit area in the region of measurement (Zeiss definition)
Fractal dimension	Describes shape or texture and determines complexity of an image
Lacunarity	Expresses patchiness or inhomogeneity of an image
Vessel perimeter index	Expresses vessel perimeter in relation to total image area
Foveal avascular zone (FAZ)	Avascular area in the center of the macula within the fovea
FAZ area	Area of the FAZ
FAZ diameter/perimeter	Diameter/Perimeter of the FAZ
FAZ circularity index	Index describing how circular the area of the FAZ is; values closer to 1 indicate higher circularity
Vessel tortuosity	Abnormal curvature of the vessels
Narrowed/dilated vessels	Morphologically obvious thinning or dilation of vessels
Branching complexity	Altered complexity of vessel branching

**Vessel density can be measured by area- or length-based measurements. Length-based measurements are more sensitive to changes in small capillaries; in area-based measurements, larger vessels have greater influence. Synonyms for vessel density: vascular/microvascular/capillary/flow density. Reprinted with permission from ref. [15].*

Table 1.
Commonly used OCT-A expressions and parameters.

3. Neuro-ophthalmological conditions

3.1 Papilledema and pseudopapilledema

Papilledema is swelling of the optic nerve head (ONH) caused by increased intracranial pressure (ICP) eventually causing stasis in axonal transport. Distinguishing it from pseudopapilledema, caused by a congenital optic disc elevation (crowded optic disc) or optic disc drusen, can be difficult based on ophthalmoscopic features alone [16]. Studies have suggested that the shape and thickness of the retinal nerve fiber layer (RNFL) around the ONH as seen on spectral-domain OCT (SD-OCT) can distinguish between ONH drusen and edema. However, SD-OCT can only show the presence of ONH drusen and cannot determine if there is also swelling present. In such cases, fluorescein dye tests can be used to determine if there is true edema present [3]. Fard *et al.* demonstrated that whole image and nasal peripapillary sector capillary densities using OCT-A had diagnostic accuracy for differentiating true and pseudo-disc swelling [16]. They showed there was a significantly lower whole image and nasal sector peripapillary capillary density of the inner retina in pseudopapilledema eyes than papilledema eyes. The peripapillary vasculature values were found to be lower in both papilledema and pseudopapilledema eyes compared to healthy eyes when analyzed using commercial machine software. However, when using their customized software, the peripapillary capillary density in papilledema eyes was not significantly different from healthy eyes (**Figure 3**). On the other hand, the peripapillary capillary density in pseudopapilledema eyes was found to be significantly lower compared to healthy eyes.

Again, the main differentiating characteristic of papilledema from other pseudo edemas (e.g., non-arteritic anterior ischemic optic neuropathy (NAION)) on ONH OCT-A is the vascular dropout observed in NAION [3]. Rougier *et al.* [10] examined the changes in the blood vessels in eyes with disc edema and found that there were changes in the capillary network around the ONH in cases of non-arteritic NAION and papillitis, while in cases of papilledema, there were dilated and tortuous superficial blood vessels without any changes in the capillary network. The study suggests that the decreased visibility of the capillary network in cases of papilledema is likely due to the swelling of the optic disc, rather than an actual lack of blood flow, and that this may be related to changes in blood flow regulation. The cases are highlighted in **Table 2** for the enhancement of clinical knowledge of the readership and the author's observation of the retrospective analysis of all such related cases are highlighted too.

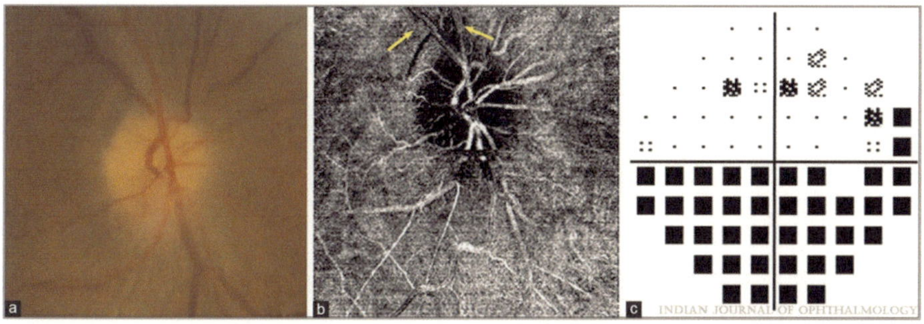

Figure 3.
Disc photograph (a) of an eye with NAION and OCT-A (b) showing superior focal loss of microvasculature (yellow arrows) and a corresponding inferior visual field defect (c). Reprinted with permission from ref. [17].

ONH Edema Type	Clinical Cases	Figures	Observations
Ischemic	A 65 years old woman with an acute visual loss of her right eye related to NAION	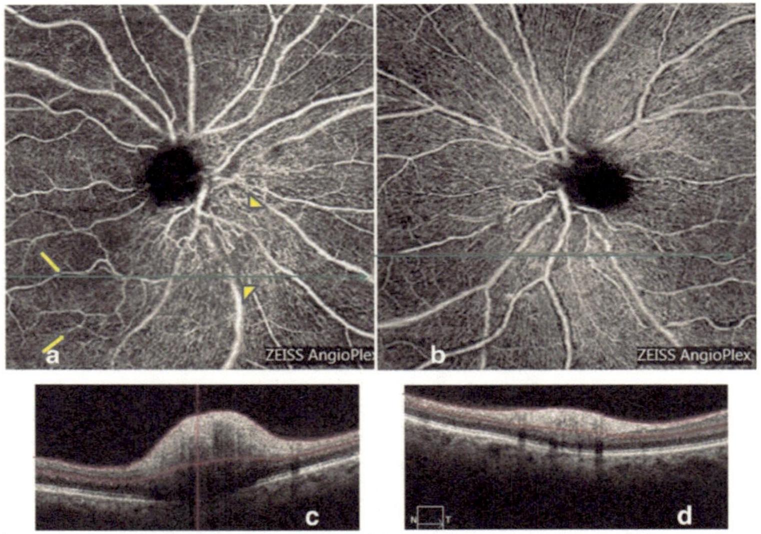 [Figure: The patient's right eye's superficial OCT-A (Angioplex©) image (a) reveals dilated capillaries that have a convoluted appearance on the nasal side of the optic disc. (arrowheads). There are some dark spots on the temporal side that represent a vascular drop out. (arrows). There is no edema in the vascular dropout area, and there is no shadowing artifact, according to the B-scan inferior to the optic disc. (c). The peripapillary network seems regular and free from vascular dropout in the healthy eye (b and d). The location and direction of the B-Scans are indicated by green arrows inside the OCT-A pictures.]	In all NAION eyes, the peripapillary network was less visible, especially around the edema area. There was some vascular dropout (arrows), displayed by dark areas. In some eyes, vascular tortuosity at the surface of the optic disc was visible (arrowheads). The global aspect was a severe disappearance of the peripapillary regular pattern.

ONH Edema Type	Clinical Cases	Figures	Observations
Inflammatory	52 years old male presenting a papillitis on the left eye related to syphilis infection	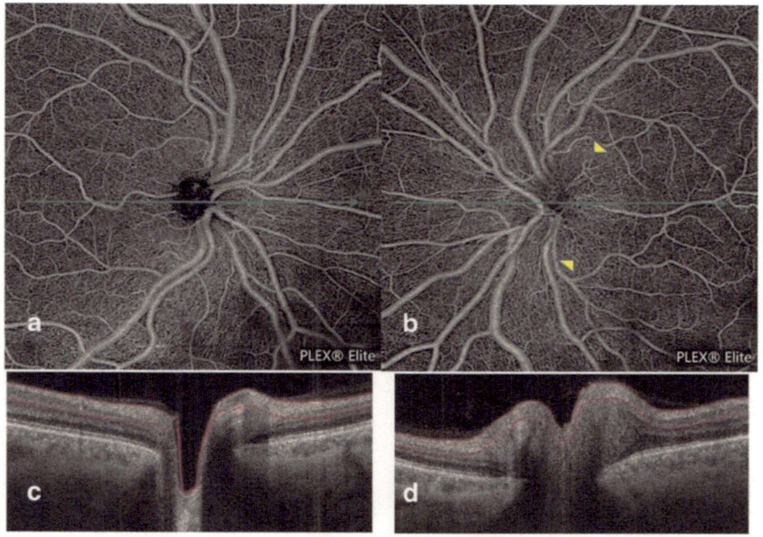 [Figure: On the left eye (b), superficial OCT-A (Plexelite) is nearly normal, and the superficial optic disc vessels are somewhat dilated. (arrowheads). There is no vascular tortuosity or dropout. The peripapillary network seems regular when compared to the healthy eye (a). OCT-B images (c and d) matching a and b]	In inflammatory optic disc edema (e.g., papillitis), no vascular dropout was present. When the ONH edema was significant, the capillaries sometimes disappeared in the edema, but they were visible above the edematous area. More often, the radial distribution of the peripapillary capillaries remained preserved, and some vascular dilation could be seen in some eyes. The global aspect was a moderate alteration of the peripapillary regular pattern.

ONH Edema Type	Clinical Cases	Figures	Observations
Papilledema	A 25 year old female presenting bilateral papilledema related to idiopathic intracranial hypertension	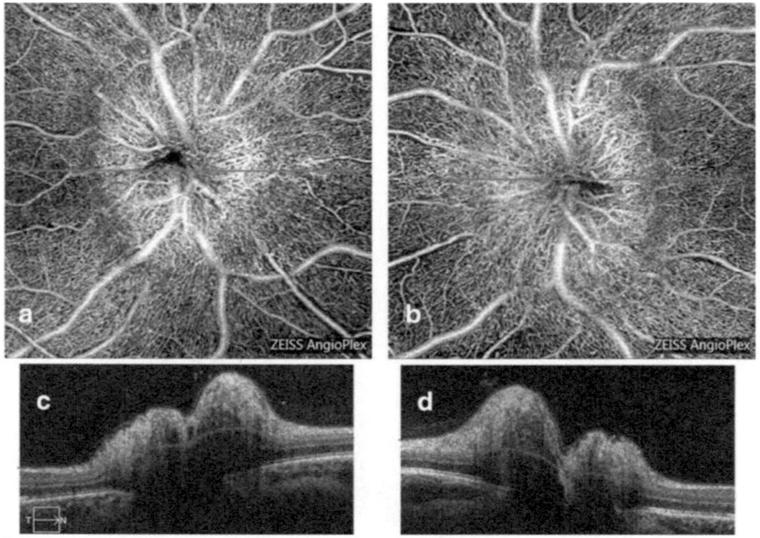[Figure: Superficial OCT-A of both eyes (a and b) taken with Angioplex showing a dilatation of the convoluted and dilated superficial optic disc arteries. The optic disc seems to be a tangled ball of vessels when viewed from all angles. (arrowheads). OCT-B scans (c and d), which correlate to (a and b)	In papilledema, the author's 12 patients had bilateral papilledema. The 13th patient presented unusual unilateral papilledema, but the opening pressure measured during the lumbar puncture confirmed the diagnosis of idiopathic intracranial hypertension. In these eyes, the radial peripapillary network was unchanged. The capillaries at the surface of the optic nerve head were dilated and tortuous like a tangled ball of vessels (arrowheads). There was no vascular dropout. The global appearance was of a bushy aspect.

Figures are reprinted with permission from ref. [10].

Table 2.
OCT-A of different kinds of optic nerve head (ONH) edema and corresponding example clinical cases.

The authors concluded that the morphological analysis of OCT-A appeared to be more beneficial than the quantification analysis in the acute phase, enabling the differentiation between the three kinds of ONH edema: ischemic, inflammatory, and papilledema [10].

Another significant application of OCT-A is in glaucoma. Studies have shown that changes in the blood vessels in the eyes, seen through OCT angiography (OCT-A), can be useful in diagnosing primary open-angle glaucoma. This is because these changes are consistent with the pathophysiology of the disease and can provide complementary information to traditional diagnostic methods. Vessel density loss associated with glaucoma can be detected by OCT-A. Peripapillary, macular, and choroidal vessel density parameters may complement visual field and structural OCT measurements in the diagnosis of glaucoma. Interested authors may refer to a separate chapter on this topic in this book [18]. OCT-A may be particularly useful in evaluating patients who are suspected of having glaucoma and in monitoring advanced cases [19, 20].

Classification	Diseases	Pathology	Epidemiology
Inflammatory	• Demyelinating optic neuritis (ON)	• Early sign of neuromyelitis optica spectrum disorder (NMOSD), multiple sclerosis (MS), or other autoimmune disorders on the spinal cord, brain, and optic nerve • Anti-aquaporin-4 (AQP4) and anti-myelin oligodendrocyte glycoprotein (MOG) auto-antibodies can be discovered • Exist subtype of no specific antibody identified	• Affecting young adults ranging from 18 to 45 years of age, with a mean age of 30–35 years • Strong female predominance • Approximate annual incidence of 5/100,000, with an estimated prevalence of 115/100,0008
Ischemic	• Non-arteritic anterior ischemic optic neuropathy (NAION)	• Non-inflammatory disease of short posterior ciliary artery • Coincidence of cardiovascular risk factors in a patient with "crowded" optic discs	• 2.3 and 10.3 per 100,000 population per year
	• Arteritic anterior ischemic optic neuropathy (AION)	• Temporal arteritis (also called giant-cell arteritis)	• About 8000 individuals per year in the United States
	• Posterior ischemic optic neuropathy (PION)	• Inadequate blood flow (ischemia) to retrobulbar portion of the optic nerve	• PION most commonly affects the elderly
Hereditary	• Leber hereditary optic neuropathy (LHON)	• Mitochondrial inherited (transmitted from mother to offspring) degeneration of RGCs and their axons	• In Northern European populations, about one in 9000 people carry one of the three primary LHON mutations

Reprinted with permission from ref. [11].

Table 3.
Different types of optic neuropathies.

3.2 Optic neuropathies

Optic neuropathies refer to a spectrum of disorders with abnormalities and dysfunction of the optic nerve [11]. **Table 3** summarizes different types of optic neuropathies and their pathology and epidemiology.

Anterior ischemic optic neuropathies (AAION) can be divided into two types: arteritic (AAION) and nonarteritic (NAION). AAION is commonly linked to giant cell arteritis, a severe form of vasculitis that affects vision. NAION, on the other hand, mainly affects individuals with cardiovascular risk factors and those with crowded optic discs [3]. NAION is the most common optic neuropathy (other than glaucoma) beyond the age of 50 years. The pathogenesis of NAION is related to vascular dysfunction and is thought to be a result of the occlusion of the short posterior ciliary arteries [17].

Studies using quantitative analysis in OCT-A (Optical Coherence Tomography Angiography) have shown that AAION has more abnormal blood vessels compared to NAION. This may be justified by the fact that AAION is characterized by more swelling of the optic disk [3]. Though there is no definite quantitative cut-off value for differentiating AAION from NAION, clinical applications of OCT-A in NAION are reported in several studies investigating the retinal vessels, choroidal vasculature, and optic disc perfusion. Karrabi *et al.* summarized different studies comparing NAION, fellow eyes, and normal eyes and interested readers may refer to it [3].

OCT-A studies have consistently shown changes in the blood vessels of patients with NAION. The most common changes include tortuous capillaries, irregularity, and loss of the peripapillary vessels, particularly in the temporal and superior sectors. Disc edema or hemorrhage can affect the signal and cause a decrease in blood flow density, which may not necessarily indicate an ischemic process but rather be a result of compressive edema or imaging artifacts. Two patterns of vasculature loss in NAION have been observed, a diffuse loss of the microvasculature network and additional sectoral choroidal vascular dropout. Decreased vessel density, which is the proportion of the measured area occupied by vessels, has been found in patients with NAION compared to healthy individuals. This reduction can be reversed and may also have prognostic values. However, it should be kept in mind that part of this vascular density reduction and its reversibility can be a result of the artifact caused by optic disc edema during the acute phase of the disease [3].

Though macular OCT-A findings in NAION are debated and controversial, there is a good correlation between perfusion and visual acuity, visual field defect, and structural changes in the ONH. The decrease in peripapillary vessel density and the location of visual field defects as well as peripapillary retinal nerve fiber layer (RNFL) thinning has been reported. The whole and temporal peripapillary vessel density was strongly correlated with visual acuity, and the dropout of the temporal peripapillary superficial retinal microvasculature was associated with visual acuity loss. OCT-A revealed hypoperfusion in the retinal pigment epithelium (RPE) and peripapillary capillaries (PPC) following NAION, especially at the level of the choroid, corresponding to both functional and structural impairments. Irreversible vascular damage can lead to a decrease in perfusion, which can negatively affect visual outcomes in selective quadrants. The temporal and superior quadrants had the most reduction in vessel density, which is consistent with the commonly identified inferonasal field defect (**Figure 3**) [3, 17].

In other types of optic neuropathy, toxic and traumatic optic neuropathy, OCT-A might not be useful and structural assessment is still superior to vascular parameters in differentiating toxic and traumatic optic neuropathies [3]. Apart from it, Montorio *et al.* [21] found that OCT-A can provide a detailed and quantitative analysis of early retinal vascular perfusion alterations over time after traumatic retinopathy, demonstrating that the impairment of the retinal microvasculature and its progressive changes over time occurred even in the absence of compromised visual acuity. Hence, OCT-A may be useful for monitoring the course of vascular changes in traumatic optic neuropathy [21].

OCT-A has been used in studying hereditary optic neuropathies (e.g., Leber's hereditary optic neuropathy or LHON) as well. First described in 1871 by Leber, LHON is a maternally inherited mitochondrial disease caused by mutations in the mitochondrial DNA that affects complex I of the oxidative phosphorylation chain [3, 22]. Yu *et al.* demonstrated that the retinal structure and the perfusion of the macular and peripapillary areas are reduced in subacute LHON, and the retinal structure and the perfusion of the peripapillary area are further reduced in chronic LHON [22].

Recently there has been growing interest in implementing OCT-A in diabetic retinopathy (DR). OCT-A has a potential role as an objective tool for evaluating diabetic retinopathy (DR) and its impact on the retina. It has been shown to visualize features associated with DR, including microaneurysms and neovascularization, and quantify changes in retinal capillaries and choriocapillaris (**Figures 4** and 5). Additionally, OCT-A can potentially detect DR earlier than what is visible on traditional fundus examination. It is a promising technology for accurately classifying DR

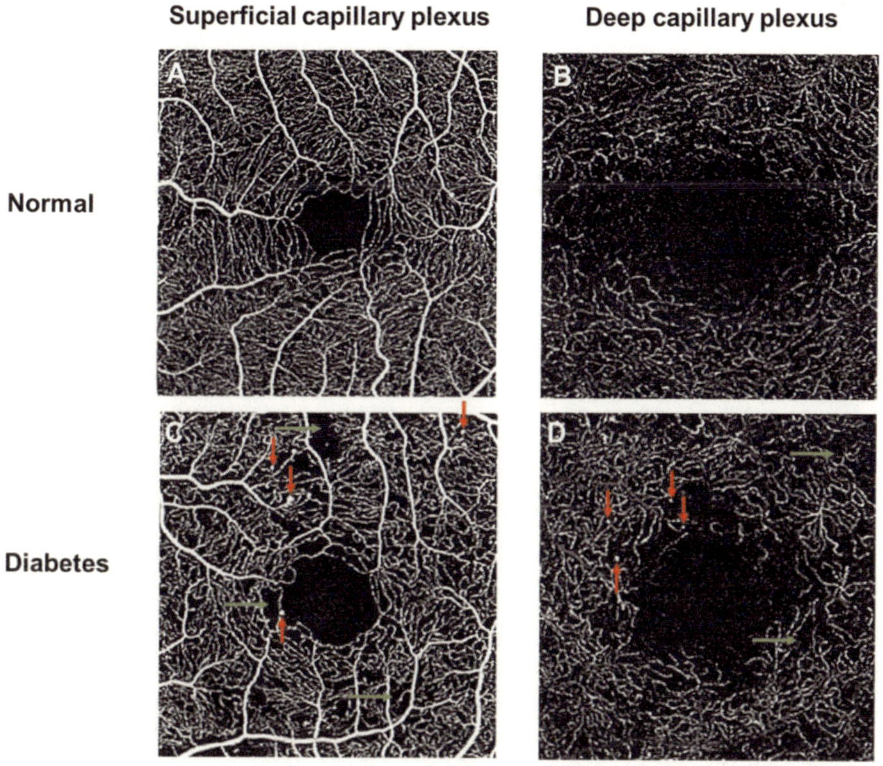

Figure 4.
A healthy control subject's optical coherence tomography angiography (OCT-A; 3 mm × 3 mm region) is shown in the top panel (A, B) and reveals a dense network of capillaries in the superficial vascular plexus, which surrounds the foveal avascular zone. A diabetic patient's OCT-A pictures (bottom panel; C, D) display vascular abnormalities in both the superficial and deep plexus layers, including microaneurysms (red arrows), capillary nonperfusion, and other vascular anomalies. (green arrows). A larger foveal avascular zone is shown. (FAZ). After the projection artifacts were eliminated, (B,D) were produced. Reprinted from ref. [12].

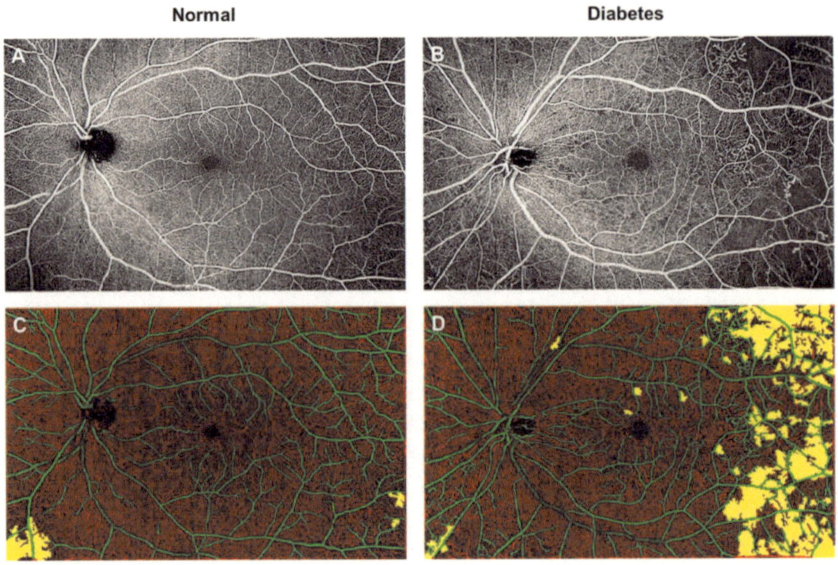

Figure 5.
Widefield optical coherence tomography angiography (OCT-A; 15 × 9 mm area; A,B) and color-coded maps showing low- or non-perfusion regions of a superficial vascular plexus in a diabetic (Right panel; C,D) and a healthy control individual (Left panel; A-C) (Right panel; B-D). In a diabetic eye, there are more areas of retinal nonperfusion, especially in the temporal regions. (D; labelled as yellow). It's imperative to keep in mind that the typical person has occasional yellow spots in the periphery. (C; labelled as yellow). Reprinted from ref. [12].

and for identifying eyes that have experienced vision loss due to diabetic macular ischemia [12, 13].

Furthermore, implementing Deep Learning (DL) in OCT-A image analysis for DR has highlighted several benefits such as early detection and progression assessment [23]. The capability of OCT-A to detect the clinical onset of DR and prediction for its progression may become valuable for the personalized management of diabetic eye disease and arguably open a new horizon of research owing to the silent epidemic of diabetes around the globe.

4. Neurological conditions with ocular manifestations

4.1 Multiple sclerosis (MS)

Multiple sclerosis (MS) is a neurodegenerative disease characterized by demyelination in CNS due to autoimmune-mediated inflammatory processes. Recently, vascular and metabolic factors are increasingly being recognized to play important roles in the neuroinflammatory mechanism of MS [4]. The optic nerve is commonly injured in MS with or without optic neuritis (ON). Optic neuritis (ON) is unilateral or bilateral inflammation of the optic nerve due to many causes, including multiple sclerosis (MS), optic neuritis associated with neuromyelitis optica (NMO), infectious, or isolated. In patients with MS, ON is the presenting symptom in 25% and occurs in 75% of cases during the disease course [3].

According to post-mortem studies, demyelinating plaques can be seen in the optic nerves of up to 99% of MS patients, making optic nerve involvement a common aspect

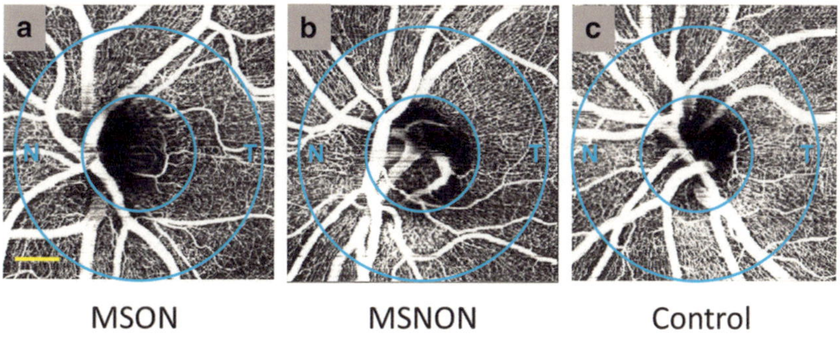

Figure 6.
Optical coherence tomography angiography (OCT-A) of the optic nerve head (ONH) in a representative Multiple Sclerosis (MS) patient. Split-spectrum amplitude decorrelation angiography (SSADA) results (N = nasal, T = temporal) show that, in comparison to (c) a healthy control example, (a) MS eyes with a history of ON (MSON) and (b) MS eyes without a history of ON (MSNON) both exhibit an apparent qualitative reduction of the ONH microvascular density in the peripapillary area (between circles), mostly in the temporal region. (c). Bar = 0.5 mm (Reprinted from ref. [5]).

of the disease process [5]. The parafoveal and ONH (**Figure 6**) flow index, a representation of relative blood flow velocity in the vasculature, was determined to be significantly lower in MS eyes with a history of ON (MSON) in comparison to eyes without a history of ON (MSNON), compared to healthy controls [5, 24, 25].

On the other hand, in the largest study of OCT-A on MS so far, Murphy *et al.* [26] showed retinal SVP densities measured by OCT-A are reduced in MS eyes in both MSON and MSNON [26]. They also found that reduced SVP densities correlate with reduced visual function, longer disease duration, and higher levels of global disability in expanded disability status scale (EDSS) and multiple sclerosis functional composite (MSFC) assessments. The group suggested that OCT-A may have additive value as a biomarker in MS, in addition to routine OCT evaluation. The suggestion is coherent with a previous study by Spain *et al.* [25] where they investigated 68 eyes from MS patients and 55 healthy eyes with OCT and OCT-A to assess the structural and vascular change in the peripapillary area. The results showed that MS patients, regardless of whether they had a history of optic neuritis (ON), had a lower ONH flow index and reduced thickness of the retinal nerve fiber layer compared to healthy control eyes. The differences were even more pronounced in MS patients with a history of ON. In comparison to their previous study with a smaller sample size, this study showed that MS patients without a history of ON had a 5.5% decrease in the ONH flow index compared to healthy controls, while MS patients with ON showed a 14.7% decrease compared to healthy controls [25].

Kleerekooper *et al.* summarized the current state of development of OCT-A in MS and some other neuroinflammatory disorders (e.g., neuromyelitis optica spectrum disorder (NMOSD)) and interested readers may refer to it [4]. Although, OCT-A gives new insight into various neuroinflammatory disorders using qualitative features of the retinal microvasculature. Prior to OCT-A being fully implemented into clinical practice, however, concerns with image quality and the creation of standardization must be resolved.

4.2 Alzheimer's disease (AD)

The neuropathology of Alzheimer's disease (AD) involves the buildup of beta-amyloid plaques and neurofibrillary tangles, which cause inflammation and neurodegeneration [8]. It is now recognized that changes in vascular remodeling also play a role in AD, dementia, and mild cognitive impairment (MCI). Due to their similar anatomic, embryonic, and physiologic characteristics, there has been evidence that the retinal vascular network is a surrogate marker of small cerebral microvascular changes [6, 8, 15, 27]. As the retinal vascular network can be observed directly in AD by OCT-A, there has been evidence of decreased retinal vascular density in AD [8, 15]. In a recently conducted systematic review by Katsimpris *et al.* summarized the OCT-A metrics in AD [6]. They found whole and parafoveal superficial venous plexus (SVP) vessel density were inversely associated with AD. This conclusion was coherent with the systematic review of Rifai *et al.* where the authors reported a significant increase in the foveal avascular zone (FAZ) area and a significant decrease in parafoveal SVP and whole SVP density in AD [27]. However, a possible limitation of OCT-A in AD is less suitable for advanced AD patients. Advanced AD patients are easily fatigued by imaging and are more prone to fixation errors [8]. OCT-A may not be useful in subjects with advanced dementia and may be most useful for patients with a new-onset or milder form of the disease. Nevertheless, though recent advances in biomedical imaging modalities like positron emission tomography (PET) have revolutionized the visualization of amyloid-β plagues presence *in vivo* in cognitively healthy individuals, it is not yet feasible as a large-scale screening procedure due to its expensive nature [6]. Compared to this, quantitative OCT-A measurements might provide cost-effective useful biomarkers for assessing the course of AD-related neurodegeneration. From a clinical perspective, it would be really beneficial if a cost-effective retinal OCT-A screening can make an early diagnosis of AD and its disease progression even before severe brain degeneration. Though it requires further study, OCT-A shows promise to develop early retinal biomarkers for pre-clinical AD pathology and its progression from dementia.

Apart from these, there has been growing interest in OCT-A-based screening for cerebral small vessel diseases (CSVD). Lee *et al.* [28] conducted a prospective cross-sectional study in the eyes of 69 (138 eyes) cognitively impaired patients to evaluate radial peripapillary capillary (RPC) network density through OCT-A and retinal nerve fiber layer (RNFL) thickness and determine their association with brain imaging markers. Among the 29 patients with amyloid-positive Alzheimer's disease-related cognitive impairment (ADCI), 25 patients with subcortical vascular cognitive impairment (SVCI), and 15 amyloid-negative cognitively normal (CN) subjects were enrolled in the study. The authors found the microvasculature of the RPC network was related to the CSVD burden. However, the RNFL thickness did not reflect cerebral neurodegeneration (**Figure** 7 and **Table 4**).

4.3 Stroke

Stroke may be defined as a neurological deficit attributed to an acute focal injury of the central nervous system (CNS) by a vascular cause, including cerebral infarction, intracerebral hemorrhage (ICH), and subarachnoid hemorrhage (SAH), and is a major cause of disability and death worldwide [29]. Of the two types of strokes: ischemic and hemorrhagic, ischemic stroke accounts for 80% of stroke cases and is characterized as an episode of neurological dysfunctions caused by focal cerebral, spinal, or retinal infarction [29, 30]. Lacunar infarctions, which are tiny infarctions (3–15 mm in diameter) in the deep perforating artery region, account for around 25% of ischemic strokes [31]. The causes of lacunar infarction and whether it differs from cortical stroke are still up for debate despite the fact that it has been acknowledged as a recognized subtype of stroke for more than 50 years. OCT-A allows the understanding of the pathophysiological processes underlying lacunar infarction in other vascular

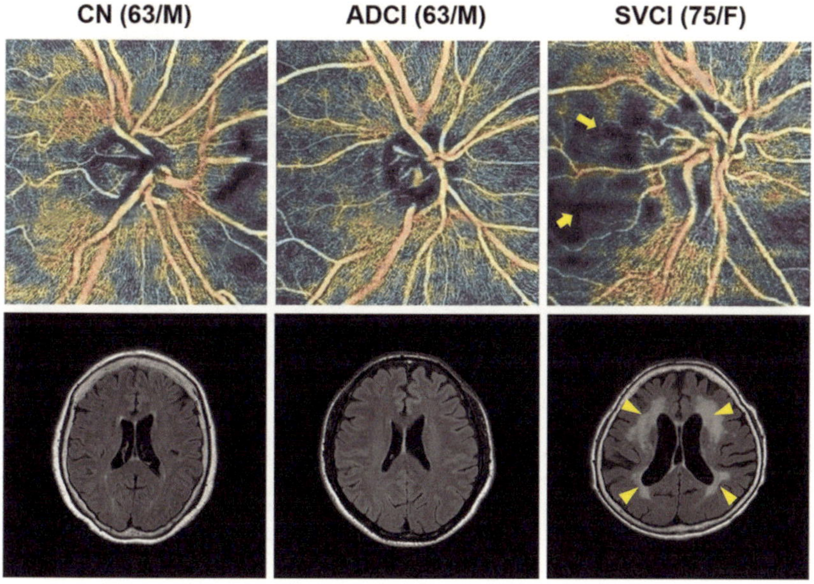

Figure 7.
Representative images according to diagnostic groups. Representative patient images of OCT-A and brain magnetic resonance imaging (MRI). Images demonstrate the subcortical vascular cognitive impairment (SVCI), the Alzheimer's disease-related cognitive impairment (ADCI), and the superficial radial peripapillary capillary network (upper row) and axial T2 fluid-attenuated inversion recovery (bottom row) of patients. The patient with SVCI has severe subcortical white matter hyperintensity and decreased peripapillary capillary network density in the temporal quadrant (arrows). (arrowheads). (Reprinted from ref. [28].)

beds, such as the retina, where small vessels can be visualized easily. Very recently, Duan *et al.* conducted the first OCT-A study and compared its metrics in lacunar and non-lacunar strokes [31]. They found retinal microvascular changes using OCT-A several years after the diagnosis of ischemic stroke. Though OCT-A is not yet established for the diagnosis of acute stroke, the modality can increase our understanding of different stroke sub-types and cerebrovascular diseases. They detected that increased FAZ axis ratio (FAR) of the deep capillary plexus (DCP) and decreased FAZ circularity (FC) of the DCP were associated with ischemic stroke. Also, decreased vascular orientation distribution (VOD) of the superficial capillary plexus (SCP) is associated with lacunar infarction compared with non-lacunar infarction.

Moreover, in a very recent study, Pachade *et al.* demonstrated that microvasculature density features from OCT-A images have the potential to be used to diagnose acute cerebral stroke from the retina. They found decreased microvasculature density, signifying a sparser vessel network, was associated with acute stroke in their study group. Using a self-supervised learning of OCT-A and fundus imaging, their diagnostic system may have a future role in relatively lower cost acute stroke diagnosis and warrants further research [7].

Apart from it, Cerebral Autosomal Dominant Arteriopathy with Subcortical Infarcts and Leukoencephalopathy (CADASIL), a rare autosomal dominant disease, is the leading cause of hereditary ischemic strokes. The vessel wall of the brain's vasculature thickens as a result of a mutation in the Notch-3 gene, leading to lumen stenosis [15]. OCT-A changes in CADASIL were found to be significantly reduced vessel density in the DCP in the macular region. When compared to the control group, there were no differences in any other macular or optic nerve head OCT-A parameters.

	ADCI, *n* = 28	SVCI, *n* = 18	CN, *n* = 14	*p* values*		
				ADCI vs. CN	SVCI vs. CN	ADCI vs. SVCI
Capillary density (CD) in the RPC network (%)						
Superior	64.15 (6.39)	60.14 (6.42)	63.16 (6.18)	1	0.121	0.033
Inferior	67.19 (7.34)	64.06 (6.07)	63.43 (7.8)	0.238	1	0.171
Temporal	45.76 (7.13)	42.34 (6.29)	48.45 (7.08)	0.471	0.001	0.048
Nasal	49.69 (5.52)	50.25 (6.29)	50.51 (5.59)	1	1	1
RNFL thickness (μm)						
Superior	129.80 (19.2)	124.19 (21.73)	126.5 (16.44)	1	1	1
Inferior	138.25 (22.21)	128.51 (19.5)	138.1 (18.51)	1	1	1
Temporal	80.48 (12.13)	76.84 (15.36)	77.79 (10.83)	1	0.906	1
Nasal	76.33 (15.64)	78.73 (11.84)	81.57 (10.99)	0.404	1	0.74

(Reprinted from ref. [28].)
**p values: after Bonferroni correction for multiple group comparison.*

Table 4.
Comparisons of capillary density in the radial peripapillary capillary (RPC) network and retinal nerve fiber layer (RNFL) thickness among the three groups.

Finally, in addition to improving our understanding of CSVD as stated in the previous section, OCT-A vascular parameters may shed light on the progression of ongoing microvascular vascular events (e.g., in hypertension, stroke, endothelial dysfunction, and inflammation) in patients.

4.4 Parkinson's disease (PD)

Previous research on the retina in Parkinson's disease (PD) patients relied solely on structural OCT scans [9]. Although OCT allows for the analysis of morphological changes in various neurological conditions, the addition of OCT-A will significantly enhance the diagnostic capabilities by enabling a closer examination of the functional and vascular components. Now, it has been established that retinal microvasculature density is associated with PD progression (**Figure 8**) [9, 32]. It was first demonstrated by Kwapong et al. [33] that OCT-A revealed decreased retinal microvascular density in early PD patients, which was later confirmed by Robbins et al. [34] too [33, 34]. In an advanced approach by Zou et al. showed combination of OCT and OCT-A in PD had better diagnostic ability than either alone, and may provide an additional biomarker for disease progression [8].

However, the limitation of OCT-A in PD is that motion artifacts increase in advanced PD patients. The possible cause is PD's cardinal motor symptoms such as tremors, bradykinesia, and rigidity, as well as neuropsychiatric symptoms like reduced attention control and bradyphrenia. The motor symptoms worsen as the disease progresses and that is why motion artifacts also increase with the duration of PD, making it difficult to obtain artifact-free OCT-A recordings, especially in the advanced stages of the disease [9]. An interesting study by Lauermann *et al.* found that motion artifacts in OCT-A images are equally common in both medicated PD patients and healthy controls [9]. However, more advanced stages of PD, indicated by longer disease duration and more severe motor symptoms, were associated with

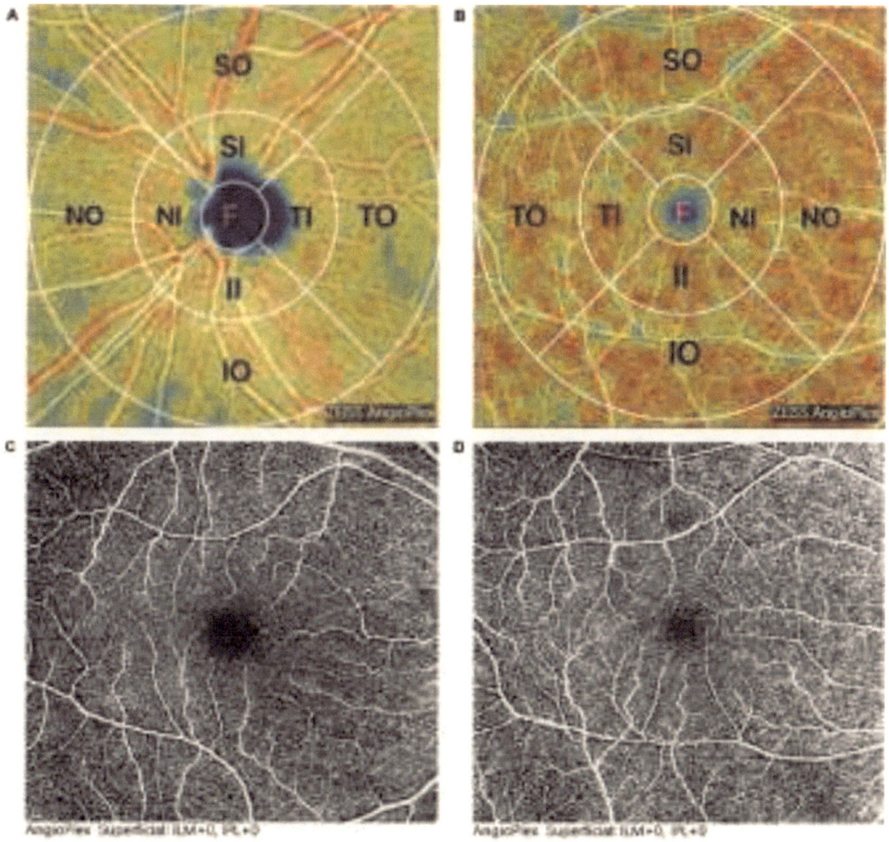

Figure 8.
Representative Optical Coherence Tomography Angiography (OCT-A) Images in PD vs control. OCT-A image and measurement of the density analysis of the superficial retinal capillary plexus (SCP). (A,B) Map of macular and peripapillary area. The inner and outer rings were divided into four quadrants: superior (SO & SI), nasal (NO & NI), inferior (IO & II), and temporal (TO & TI). (C,D) Foveal avascular zone (FAZ) area was significantly decreased in patients with Parkinson's disease (PD) (D) compared to healthy controls (HC) (C). (Reprinted from ref. [32].)

higher levels of motion artifacts. Thus, caution and expertise are necessary when evaluating the quality and interpreting the results of OCT-A images, particularly in the advanced stages of PD. More importantly, the authors suggest that as like as MRI scans are evaluated by specialized radiologists or neuroradiologists to ensure accurate results for clinical interpretation by other departments. Specialized eye clinics should create and assess OCT-A recordings and then provide the revised results to non-specialist colleagues for clinical use to mitigate such caveats. Nevertheless, OCT-A has opened a new avenue of research in early diagnosis, and disease progression from micro-perfusion changes in PD patients.

5. Conclusion

Optical Coherence Tomography Angiography (OCT-A) has emerged as a powerful tool in imaging microvasculature in different neuro-ophthalmological and central nervous system disorders. With its unique capability to provide detailed microvascular architecture, it has contributed to the diagnosis, monitoring progression, and prognosis of various conditions such as optic neuropathies, papilledema, glaucoma, multiple sclerosis, Alzheimer's disease, Parkinson's disease, different cerebral small vessel diseases, and stroke. Despite the current limitations, the future of OCT-A in neuro-ophthalmology and neurology is promising, as ongoing research continues to explore its potential applications, overcome its challenges, and further advance its capabilities.

Author details

Mobin Ibne Mokbul
Dhaka Medical College Hospital, Dhaka, Bangladesh

*Address all correspondence to: mobin.dmc@gmail.com

References

[1] Huang D, Swanson EA, Lin CP, Schuman JS, Stinson WG, Chang W, et al. Optical coherence tomography. Science. 1991;**254**(5035):1178-1181. DOI: 10.1126/science.1957169

[2] Ibne MM. Optical coherence tomography: Basic concepts and applications in neuroscience research. Journal of Medical Engineering. 2017; **2017**:3409327. DOI: 10.1155/2017/3409327 Epub 2017 Oct 29

[3] Karrabi N, Hooshmandi S, Amirabadi A, Roshandel D, Hassanpour K, Pakravan M. The role of optical coherence tomography angiography in optic nerve head Edema: A narrative review. Journal of Ophthalmology. 2022;**2022**:5823345. DOI: 10.1155/2022/5823345

[4] Kleerekooper I, Houston S, Dubis AM, Trip SA, Petzold A. Optical coherence tomography angiography (OCTA) in multiple sclerosis and neuromyelitis optica spectrum disorder. Frontiers in Neurology. 2020;**11**:604049. DOI: 10.3389/fneur.2020.604049

[5] Wang L, Murphy O, Caldito NG, Calabresi PA, Saidha S. Emerging applications of optical coherence tomography angiography (OCTA) in neurological research. Eye and Vision (London, England). 2018;**5**:11. DOI: 10.1186/s40662-018-0104-3

[6] Katsimpris A, Karamaounas A, Sideri AM, Katsimpris J, Georgalas I, Petrou P. Optical coherence tomography angiography in Alzheimer's disease: A systematic review and meta-analysis. Eye (London, England). 2022;**36**(7):1419-1426. DOI: 10.1038/s41433-021-01648-1

[7] Pachade S, Coronado I, Abdelkhaleq R, Yan J, Salazar-Marioni S, Jagolino A, et al. Detection of stroke with retinal microvascular density and self-supervised learning using OCT-A and fundus imaging. Journal of Clinical Medicine. 2022;**11**(24):7408. DOI: 10.3390/jcm11247408

[8] Yoon SP, Grewal DS, Thompson AC, Polascik BW, Dunn C, Burke JR, et al. Retinal microvascular and neurodegenerative changes in Alzheimer's disease and mild cognitive impairment compared with control participants. Ophthalmology Retina. 2019;**3**(6):489-499. DOI: 10.1016/j.oret.2019.02.002

[9] Lauermann JL, Sochurek JAM, Plöttner P, Alten F, Kasten M, Prasuhn J, et al. Applicability of optical coherence tomography angiography (OCTA) imaging in Parkinson's disease. Scientific Reports. 2021;**11**(1):5520. DOI: 10.1038/s41598-021-84862-x

[10] Rougier MB, Le Goff M, Korobelnik JF. Optical coherence tomography angiography at the acute phase of optic disc edema. Eye and Vision (London, England). 2018;**5**:15. DOI: 10.1186/s40662-018-0109-y

[11] Tan S, Yao Y, Yang Q, Yuan XL, Cen LP, Ng TK. Diversified treatment options of adult stem cells for optic neuropathies. Cell Transplantation. 2022;**31**:9636897221123512. DOI: 10.1177/09636897221123512

[12] Chua J, Sim R, Tan B, Wong D, Yao X, Liu X, et al. Optical coherence tomography angiography in diabetes and diabetic retinopathy. Journal of Clinical Medicine. 2020;**9**(6):1723. DOI: 10.3390/jcm9061723

[13] Sun Z, Yang D, Tang Z, Ng DS, Cheung CY. Optical coherence

tomography angiography in diabetic retinopathy: An updated review. Eye (London, England). 2021;**35**(1):149-161. DOI: 10.1038/s41433-020-01233-y Epub 2020 Oct 24

[14] Zhang Q, Huang Y, Zhang T, Kubach S, An L, Laron M, et al. Wide-field imaging of retinal vasculature using optical coherence tomography-based microangiography provided by motion tracking. Journal of Biomedical Optics. 2015;**20**(6):066008. DOI: 10.1117/1.JBO.20.6.066008

[15] Augustin AJ, Atorf J. The value of optical coherence tomography angiography (OCT-A) in neurological diseases. Diagnostics (Basel, Switzerland). 2022;**12**(2):468. DOI: 10.3390/diagnostics12020468

[16] Fard MA, Sahraiyan A, Jalili J, Hejazi M, Suwan Y, Ritch R, et al. Optical coherence tomography angiography in papilledema compared with Pseudopapilledema. Investigative Ophthalmology & Visual Science. 2019; **60**(1):168-175. DOI: 10.1167/iovs.18-25453

[17] Gandhi U, Chhablani J, Badakere A, Kekunnaya R, Rasheed MA, Goud A, et al. Optical coherence tomography angiography in acute unilateral nonarteritic anterior ischemic optic neuropathy: A comparison with the fellow eye and with eyes with papilledema. Indian Journal of Ophthalmology. 2018;**66**(8):1144-1148. DOI: 10.4103/ijo.IJO_179_18

[18] Kooner K, Rehman M, Suresh S, Buchanan E, Albdour M, Zuberi H. The role of optical coherence tomography angiography in glaucoma. IntechOpen; 2023. Available from: https://www.intechopen.com/online-first/86505 [Retrieved March 23, 2023]

[19] WuDunn D, Takusagawa HL, Sit AJ, Rosdahl JA, Radhakrishnan S, Hoguet A, et al. OCT angiography for the diagnosis of glaucoma: A report by the American academy of ophthalmology. Ophthalmology. 2021;**128**(8):1222-1235. DOI: 10.1016/j.ophtha.2020.12.027 Epub 2021 Feb 23

[20] Rao HL, Pradhan ZS, Suh MH, Moghimi S, Mansouri K, Weinreb RN. Optical Coherence Tomography Angiography in Glaucoma. Journal of Glaucoma. 2020 Apr;**29**(4):312-321. DOI: 10.1097/IJG.0000000000001463. PMID: 32053551; PMCID: PMC7117982

[21] Montorio D, D'Andrea L, Cennamo G. Retinal vascular features in ocular blunt trauma by optical coherence tomography angiography. Journal of Clinical Medicine. 2020;**9**(10):3329. DOI: 10.3390/jcm9103329

[22] Yu J, Xu H, Huang Y, Gu R, Zong Y, Zhu H, et al. Changes in retinal perfusion in Leber's hereditary optic neuropathy: An optical coherence tomography-angiography study. Ophthalmic Research. 2021;**64**(5):863-870. DOI: 10.1159/000518185 Epub 2021 Jul 9

[23] Guo Y, Camino A, Wang J, Huang D, Hwang TS, Jia Y. MEDnet, a neural network for automated detection of avascular area in OCT angiography. Biomedical Optics Express. 2018;**9**(11): 5147-5158. DOI: 10.1364/BOE.9.005147

[24] Wang X, Jia Y, Spain R, Potsaid B, Liu JJ, Baumann B, et al. Optical coherence tomography angiography of optic nerve head and parafovea in multiple sclerosis. The British Journal of Ophthalmology. 2014;**98**(10):1368-1373. DOI: 10.1136/bjophthalmol-2013-304547 Epub 2014 May 15

[25] Spain RI, Liu L, Zhang X, Jia Y, Tan O, Bourdette D, et al. Optical

coherence tomography angiography enhances the detection of optic nerve damage in multiple sclerosis. The British Journal of Ophthalmology. 2018;**102**(4): 520-524. DOI: 10.1136/bjophthalmol-2017-310477 Epub 2017 Aug 16

[26] Murphy OC, Kwakyi O, Iftikhar M, Zafar S, Lambe J, Pellegrini N, et al. Alterations in the retinal vasculature occur in multiple sclerosis and exhibit novel correlations with disability and visual function measures. Multiple Sclerosis (Houndmills, Basingstoke, England). Investigative Ophthalmology & Visual Science. 2020;**26**(7):815-828. DOI: 10.1177/1352458519845116

[27] Rifai OM, McGrory S, Robbins CB, Grewal DS, Liu A, Fekrat S, et al. The application of optical coherence tomography angiography in Alzheimer's disease: A systematic review. Alzheimer's & Dementia (Amsterdam, Netherlands). 2021;**13**(1):e12149. DOI: 10.1002/dad2.12149

[28] Lee JY, Kim JP, Jang H, Kim J, Kang SH, Kim JS, et al. Optical coherence tomography angiography as a potential screening tool for cerebral small vessel diseases. Alzheimer's Research & Therapy. 2020;**12**(1):73. DOI: 10.1186/s13195-020-00638-x

[29] Sacco RL, Kasner SE, Broderick JP, Caplan LR, Connors JJ, Culebras A, et al. An updated definition of stroke for the 21st century: A statement for healthcare professionals from the American Heart Association/American Stroke Association. Stroke. 2013;**44**(7): 2064-2089. DOI: 10.1161/STR.0b013e318296aeca Epub 2013 May 7. Erratum in: Stroke. 2019;50(8): e239

[30] Boursin P, Paternotte S, Dercy B, Sabben C, Maïer B. Sémantique, épidémiologie et sémiologie des accidents vasculaires cérébraux [Semantics, epidemiology and semiology of stroke]. Soins French. 2018;**63**(828): 24-27. DOI: 10.1016/j.soin.2018.06.008

[31] Duan H, Xie J, Zhou Y, Zhang H, Liu Y, Tang C, et al. Characterization of the retinal microvasculature and FAZ changes in ischemic stroke and its different types. Translational Vision Science & Technology. 2022;**11**(10):21. DOI: 10.1167/tvst.11.10.21

[32] Xu B, Wang X, Guo J, Xu H, Tang B, Jiao B, et al. Retinal microvascular density was associated with the clinical progression of Parkinson's disease. Frontiers in Aging Neuroscience. 2022; **14**:818597. DOI: 10.3389/fnagi.2022.818597

[33] Kwapong WR, Ye H, Peng C, Zhuang X, Wang J, Shen M, et al. Retinal microvascular impairment in the early stages of Parkinson's disease. Investigative Ophthalmology & Visual Science. Investigative Ophthalmology & Visual Science. 2018;**59**(10):4115-4122. DOI: 10.1167/iovs.17-23230

[34] Robbins CB, Thompson AC, Bhullar PK, Koo HY, Agrawal R, Soundararajan S, et al. Characterization of retinal microvascular and choroidal structural changes in Parkinson disease. JAMA Ophthalmology. 2021;**139**(2): 182-188. DOI: 10.1001/jamaophthalmol.2020.5730 Erratum in: JAMA Ophthalmol. 2021 Feb 1;139(2):256

Section 3

Optical Coherence Tomography and Miscellaneous

Chapter 9

Study and Analysis of Fluid Filled Abnormalities in Retina Using OCT Images

Sumathi Manickam, I. Rexiline Sheeba and K. Venkatraman

Abstract

Visual impairment is one of the most regularly happening infections in human. The reason being variation from the normal in the different layers of retina because of strange measure of liquid either abundance aggregation or shortage. This paper targets recognizing and assessing the different abnormalities that could be earlier stages to visual deficiency. The proposed target is achieved by means of implementation using Digital Image Processing Technique, starting from preprocessing to classification at various stages. Not restricting to binary classification as normal or abnormal, the proposed system also extends its capacity to classify the input image as Cystoid Macular Edema (CME), Choroidal Neo Vascular Membrane (CNVM), Macular Hole (MH) and normal images. The preprocessing methodology implemented filters to remove the speckle noises which are most common in ultrasound-based imaging system. Random forest classifier was utilized for classifying the input features and also seems to be promising on par with the various existing methodologies.

Keywords: classifiers, ophthalmic imaging, optical coherence tomography, retinal disorders, fluid filled abnormalities

1. Introduction

Biomedical Imaging and automations in medicine has become an emerging field due to the need of precision, accuracy and storage/retrieval capability of the data being handled. Automations in the field of ophthalmology has also proven to be an emerging need of the hour as more accurate diagnosis of small changes in the retinal layers shall prevent the vision impairment. Such variations are commonly initiated owing the alterations in fluid pattern of the retinal coverings. The fluid may become excess or deficit based on the specified abnormality and due to this the patient may suffer a loss of vision. In order to identify this fluid pattern more accurately ultrasound-based imaging modality, namely, developing imaging techniques such as Optical Coherence Tomography (OCT) Ghastly Domain Optical Coherence Tomography (SD-OCT) mentioned in [1], which unmistakably differentiates numerous infections in different layers of the retina [2]. An inner layer of an eye is Retina which changes over the occurrence bright flag into neural sign, which are conveyed to the mind. It comprises of different shades, poles and cones are in charge of blurred light and shading dreams individually. Retina has a few layers of neurotic and physiological significance. Some harms in the retina layers lead to few more hazard variations from the norm including vision loss. Prior examination of OCT Images focused on separation of Intraretinal layers [3–12], division of fluid engaged layers, [13, 14] and optical circle is a fundamental one.

Medical Image Processing classification assumes a remarkable work towards familiar proof and outcome of variations are observed from the model in different imaging modalities. OCT employs ultrasound waves as a source and transceives the corresponding pictures of different layers of retina [15]. OCT is utilized in 3D reconstructible picture of retina which is required for better comprehension of real investigation, liquid-based variation from the norm. Priori stages to visual deficiency incorporate modifications in the liquid example of the different retinal layers. Scarcely any such anomalies are cystoids macular edema (CME), wherein the macular layer gets gathered with abundance of liquids, Choroidal Neo Vascular Membrane (CNVM), a fresh recruits' vessels are framed and liquid substance winds up more in the Choroidal layer, and Macular Hole (MH), wherein the macular layer progresses towards becoming shortfall of liquids. Various methodologies and implementation of the proposed system is explained in the below section.

2. Methods and materials

The overall flow diagram of the entire methodology could be clearly understood from **Figure 1**.

Images are acquired using SD OCT Device in digital format and provided as input to our system. Image inputs are exposed to preprocessing which includes grayscale conversion and noise removal. OCT practices ultrasound as a wellspring of imaging, the pictures are increasingly inclined to spot commotions, in nature these are multiplicative [16–20]. So as to dispense with/limit these commotions, homomorphic channels were utilized to kill the spot clamors. In spite of the fact that different channels are available. In the wake of preprocessing, so as to seclude the retinal layers, various methodology of division [19–22] is listed out. This assurance the retinal layers of intrigue remain disengaged from the repetitive foundation for additional handling of the image. This dynamic division calculation, the Gradient Vector stream calculation of division in the framework of projected and assessed. The division calculation figures the dissemination of slope vectors of dim level or paired edge map which is gotten from the info preprocessed picture. Therefore, the yield is normal give an unmistakable perspective on the obligatory retinal layers with liquid founded irregularities as opposed to considering the whole picture information for further preparing.

Different highlights of the divided picture were extricated among which they chose highlights are Skewness, Entropy, Variance and Energy which are the factual highlights which are utilized as info information in characterization of the pictures as typical and strange. Critical contrasts could be found in the highlights of ordinary and unusual pictures and consequently these are utilized in further arrangement. (A variance image, an image of variances that is the squares of the standard deviations, of input or output images). If a variance set is delivered, all pixel values of the variance image must be the pixels of inset which may have any value.

The separated highlights are part for preparing and testing/approval of the classifiers in a proportion of 3:1 for accomplishing a superior generally speaking

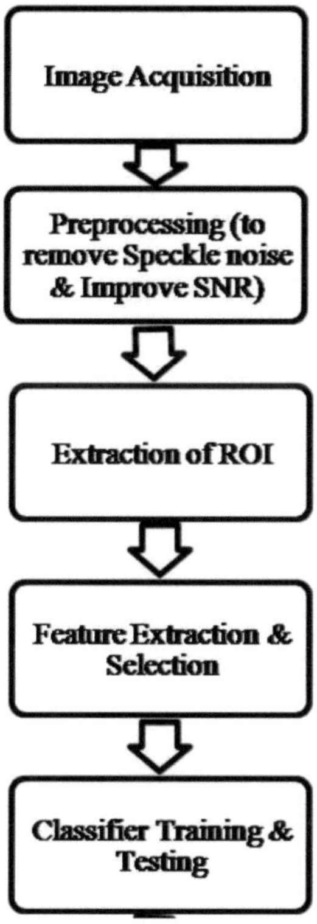

Figure 1.
Proposed methodology.

execution of the classifiers. The highlights are exhibited to Random Forest Classifier so as to get the yield in paired structure either as Normal or Abnormal. Random Forest Classifier assesses the information include into various classes and plays out a democratic check to decide the most extreme likelihood in having a place of the information highlight vector. The classifier checks for the lion's share casting a ballot under each woodland and characterizes the info occurrence dependent on the most extreme votes. Random forest includes of a huge number of discrete choice trees that work as a congregation.

Endless supply of the component information, above all clarified classifiers, the yields of the equivalent are arranged to recognize untrue positive, True negative, genuine positive and untrue negative [23, 24]. From these qualities' affectability, explicitness and thus the general framework precision/execution is being assessed for every one of the classifiers independently and this outcome is utilized to recognize the best classifier among the proposed calculations.

3. Result

The new proposed procedure was realized for 114 Images which were obtained from Topcon and Zeiss OCT gadgets. Among the accessible dataset of 27 Normal Images and 87 Abnormal Images, in absolute 70 level of the pictures were used for preparing and 30 rate where utilized for testing and validations. Right off the bat the

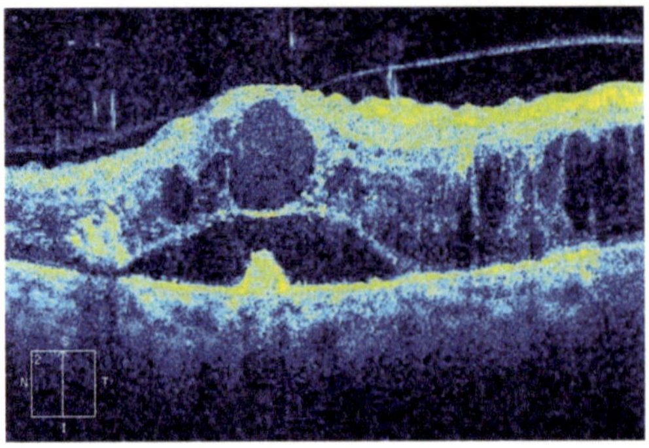

Figure 2.
Input image.

picture changes over gray scale and exposed to preprocessing utilizing various filters for evacuation of speckles. While the original input image and gray level image could be seen in **Figures 2** and **3** respectively, the outputs of various filters evaluated is shown below in **Figure 4**.

When most of the filters just average the data instead of removing the speckles, the computational results show that Homomorphic wiener filter is comparatively better, as the filter is converting the multiplicative noises into additive and hence noise removal is much efficient.

Preprocessed images are exposed to segmentation utilizing Gradient Vector Flow calculation. From the segmented image, different highlights like, Skewness, Entropy, Energy, and Variance were extricated and these highlights spoke to have a critical striking distinction among the ordinary and anomalous pictures. With these highlights as features to the classifiers, the data is being presented to the random forest network classifier whose various statistical values are being tabulated in **Tables 1** and **2**. The various parameters of statistics include True Positives, True Negatives, Untrue Positives and Untrue Negatives, Specificity, Accuracy, and Sensitivity.

From the general outcomes it is reasonable that Random Forest classifier is by all accounts equally more hopeful than different classifiers. These results seem to be similarly efficient and comparable with the previous related works.

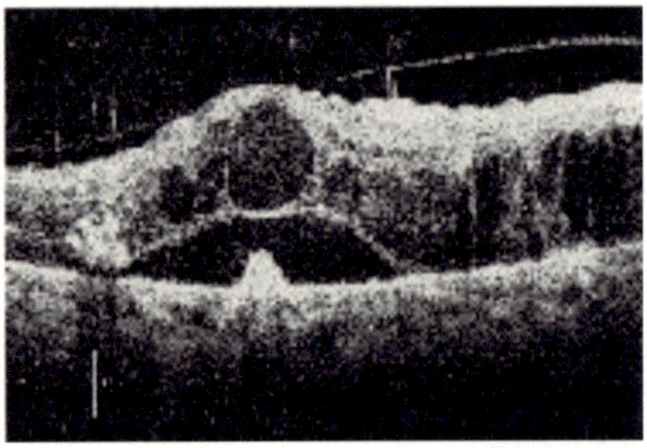

Figure 3.
Grayscale image.

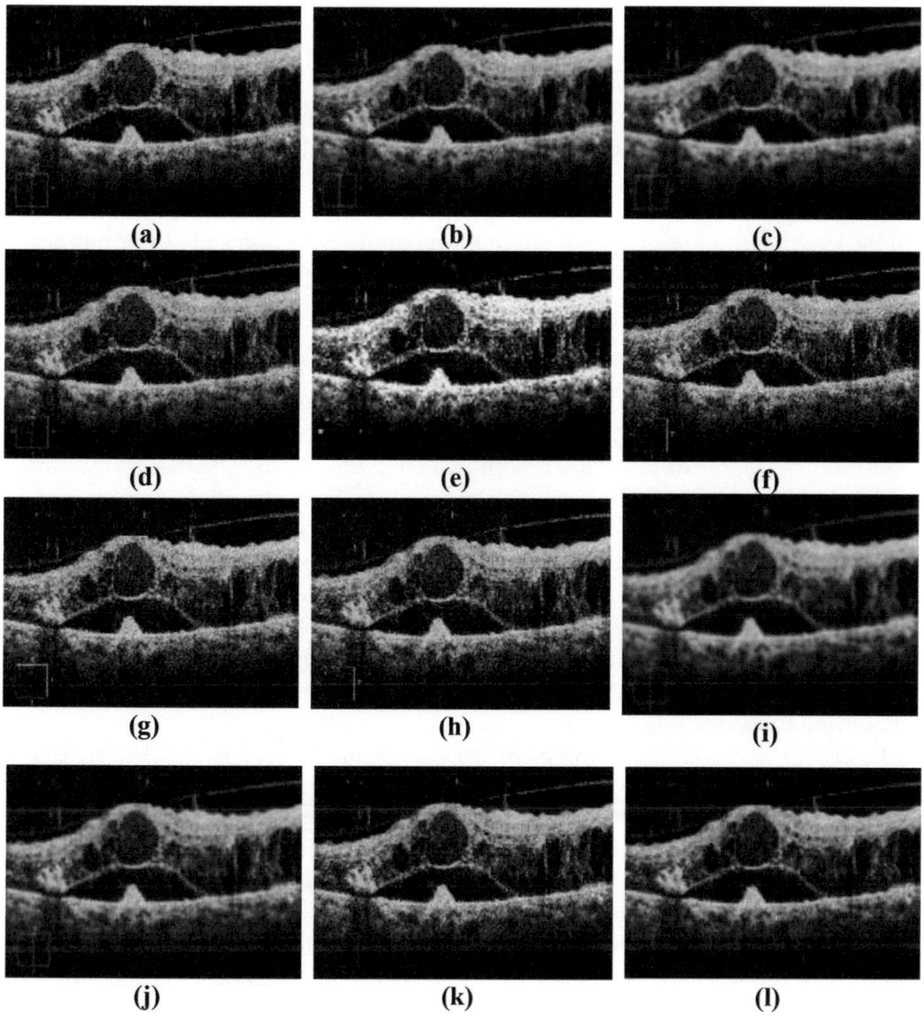

Figure 4.
*Output of various speckle reduction filters. (a) Mean filter 3*3, (b) mean filter 5*5, (c) mean filter 7*7, (d) frost filter, (e) adaptive smoothing filters, (f) Gaussian filters 3*3, (g) Gaussian filters 5*5, (h) Gaussian filters 7*7, (i) bilateral filters, (j) anisotropic diffusion filters, (k) homomorphic wiener filters 3*3, (l) homomorphic wiener filters 5*5.*

Condition	TP (%)	FP (%)	FN (%)	TN (%)
Abnormal	87.50	12.50	96.15	3.85
Normal	96.15	3.85	87.50	12.50

Table 1.
Performance output of random Forest classifier.

Classifier	Sensitivity	Specificity	Accuracy
Random Forest	87.50	96.15	91.82

Table 2.
Performance analysis of overall system.

4. Discussion

The Random Forest classifier seems to be comparatively efficient which is shown in the obtained results, when compared to the other classifiers, comparing to the earlier related works [25–27], the proposed system seems to be equally efficient towards classifying the input image as abnormal and normal. The overall system parameters like specificity, sensitivity, and accuracy seems to be more hopeful when compared with the existing methodologies as cited. By expanding the range of abnormalities and also identifying age related disorders can be further enhanced.

5. Conclusion

The proposed framework, and calculations of arrangement, is by all accounts proficient. The degree of precision accomplished demonstrates that the framework can likewise be used for useful ramifications. The effectiveness of the proposed classifier frameworks should be assessed for explicit variation from the norm-based arrangement like Cystoid Macular Edema, Choroidal Neo Vascular Membrane, Epi Retinal Membrane, Macular Hole, Age related Macular Degeneration in future, in view of the real execution could be precisely examined in detail. On definite issue-based order study, the created framework can likewise be coordinated with the OCT gadgets progressively to consequently remark on the pictures that are given as the contribution to the framework.

The developed system was implemented and evaluated with MATLAB and the validation of the system was done with reference to Ophthalmologists. The comments of the ophthalmologists on the proposed system is attached. Though the overall accuracy of the system matches the earlier works, significant improvisation could be seen with the number of abnormalities that had been included in the process of classification. With overall system accuracy of around 91.65% the proposed system is significantly in match with the existing systems. The accuracy, sensitivity, specificity and Youden's index are acceptable for the system proposed and has been cross validated for its performance by Ophthalmologists and found to be satisfactory. The obtained results in terms of accuracy of 91.65% are closer with the related works whose accuracies are closer to the values obtained by the proposed system Reza Rasti et al. [16]. The obtained performance metrics shows that the acquired accuracy is remarkably higher than the works of Philipp Seebock et al. of 81.4%, which focused to limited abnormalities. The comparison could be understood from the representation in **Table 3**.

Earlier works focused on morphological parameters alone which restricted the number of disorders taken into consideration for categorization. Apart from the morphological parameters of bulkiness, compactness and convexity, the evaluated system also used Zernike moments which is widely varying feature for the disorders

Metrics	Proposed	Philipp Seebock et al.
Accuracy	91.65%	81.4%
Number of disorders	3	1

Table 3.
Comparison of performance.

DOI: http://dx.doi.org/10.5772/intechopen.109646

chosen. The overall number of features considered has been comparatively reduced with significant accuracy, thereby optimizing the features used for the process of classification. Based on the excess or deficit of fluids in the retinal layers, the overall features also varied accordingly, so as to enable the classifier to remain comparatively more accurate for the proposed system. Zernike moments are most commonly used shape descriptors and were hence used for the proposed application, in order to detect the shape-based changes that occur in retina due to accumulation or lack of fluid within the retinal layers. The classifier that has been used is a basic supervised classifier, yet more appropriate for the application proposed. The average Youden 's Index shows that the algorithm proposed is reliable in retinal analysis and could be used in automated analysis of OCT Image analysis. The proposed system could be further extended for other disorders in retina and integrated with OCT Device as an additional software for instantaneous evaluation of the retinal disorders and the therapeutic efficiencies. The developed system is promising for the selected application and has been evaluated with comparatively higher number of input samples, which restricted its evaluation until the process of segmentation and did not focus on classification further. The overall performance indices are also satisfactory and matchable with the existing results derived from similar works as evaluated by the Ophthalmologist. The developed system has also covered a significant number of fluid related disorders which are caused due to excessive or deficit fluids within the layers of retina. As OCT is an efficient tool for detection of prior stages of blindness, the proposed algorithm remains an expert system for earlier identification and accurate evaluation of the retinal fluid volumes.

Author details

Sumathi Manickam*, I. Rexiline Sheeba and K. Venkatraman
Sathyabama Institute of Science and Technology, Chennai, Tamilnadu, India

*Address all correspondence to: sumathi.ece@sathyabama.ac.in

References

[1] Wojtkowski M, Leitgeb R, Kowalczyk A, Bajraszewski T, Fercher AF. In vivo human retinal imaging by Fourier domain optical coherence tomography. Journal of Biomedical Optics. 2002;7(3):457-463

[2] de Boer JF, Cense B, Park BH, Pierce MC, Tearney GJ, Bouma BE. Improved signal-to-noise ratio in spectral-domain compared with time-domain optical coherence tomography. Optics Letters. 2003;**28**(21):2067-2069

[3] Yazdanpanah A, Hamarneh G, Smith B, Sarunic M. Intra-retinal layer segmentation in optical coherence tomography using an active contour approach. In: Medical Image Computing and Computer-Assisted Intervention — MICCAI 2009, Part II. Vol. 5762, LNCS. New York: Springer; 2009. pp. 649-656

[4] Koozekanani D, Boyer K, Roberts C. Retinal thickness measurements from optical coherence tomography using a Markovboundary model. IEEE Transactions on Medical Imaging. 2001;**20**(9):900-916

[5] Ishikawa H, Stein DM, Wollstein G, Beaton S, Fujimoto JG, Schuman JS. Macular segmentation with optical coherence tomography. Investigative Ophthalmology & Visual Science. 2005;**46**(6):2012-2017

[6] Cabrera Fernández D, Salinas HM, Puliafito CA. Automateddetection of retinal layer structures on optical coherence tomographyimages. Optics Express. 2005;**13**(25):10200-10216

[7] Shahidi M, Wang Z, Zelkha R. Quantitative thickness measurementof retinal layers imaged by optical coherence tomography. American Journal of Ophthalmology. 2005;**139**(6):1056-1061

[8] Baroni M, Fortunato P, Torre AL. Towards quantitative analysisof retinal features in optical coherence tomography. Medical Engineering & Physics. 2007;**29**(4):432-441

[9] Fuller A, Zawadzki R, Choi S, Wiley D, Werner J, Hamann B. Segmentation of three-dimensional retinal image data. IEEE Transactions on Visualization and Computer Graphics. 2007;**13**(6):1719-1726

[10] Garvin MK, Abràmoff MD, Kardon R, Russell SR, Wu X, Sonka M. Intraretinal layer segmentation of macular optical coherencetomography images using optimal 3-D graph search. IEEE Transactions on Medical Imaging. 2008;**27**(10):1495-1505

[11] Garvin MK, Abràmoff MD, Wu X, Russell SR, Burns TL, Sonka M. Automated 3-D intraretinal layer segmentation of macularspectral-domain optical coherence tomography images. IEEE Transactions on Medical Imaging. 2009;**28**(9):1436-1447

[12] Zhihong H, Niemeijer M, Abràmoff MD, Garvin MK. Multimodal retinal vessel segmentation from spectral-domain optical coherence tomography and fundus photography. IEEE Transactions on Medical Imaging. 2012;**31**(10):1900-1911

[13] Fernández DC. Delineating fluid-filled region boundaries in optical coherence tomography images of the retina. IEEE Transactions on Medical Imaging. 2005;**24**(8):929-945

[14] Quellec G, Lee K, Dolejsi M, Garvin MK, Abramoff MD, Sonka M.

Three-dimensional analysis of retinal layer texture: Identification of fluid-filled regions in SD-OCT of the macula. IEEE Transactions on Medical Imaging. 2010;**29**(6):1321-1330

[15] Ganjee R, Moghaddam ME, Nourinia R. Automatic segmentation of abnormal capillary non perfusion regions in optical coherence tomography angiography images using marker-controlled watershed algorithm||. Journal of Biomedical Optics. 2018;**23**(9):096006-1-096006-16

[16] Rasti R, Rabbani H, Mehridehnavi A, Hajizadeh F. Macular OCT classification using a multi-scale convolutional neural network ensemble||. IEEE Transactions on Medical Imaging. 2018;**37**(4):1024-1034

[17] Venkatraman K, Sumathi M. Review of optical coherence tomography image analysis for retinal disorders. International Journal of Pharmacology & Technology. 2014;**6**(2):2967-2980

[18] Sun S, Guo Q, Lei B, Gao BZ, Dong F. Image denoising algorithm based on contourlet transform for optical coherence tomography heart tube image. IET Image Processing. 2013;**7**(5):442-450

[19] Avanaki MRN, Cernat R, Tadrous PJ, Tatla T, Podoleanu AG, Ali Hojjatoleslami S. Spatial compounding algorithm for speckle reduction of dynamic focus OCT images. IEEE Photonics Technology Letters. 2013;**25**(15):1439-1442

[20] Manojlovic LM. Novel method for optical coherence tomography resolution enhancement. IEEE Journal of Quantum Electronics. 2011;**47**(3):340-347

[21] Wilkins GR, Houghton OM, Oldenburg AL. Automated segmentation of intrarentinal cystoid fluid in optical coherence tomography. IEEE Transactions on Biomedical Engineering. 2013;**59**(4):1109-1114

[22] Wang C, Wang YX, Li Y. Automatic choroidal layer segmentation using markov random field and level set method. IEEE Journal of Biomedical and Health Informatics. 2017;**21**(6):1694-1702

[23] Maria A. Measures of diagnostic accuracy: Basic definitions. EJIFCC. 2009;**19**(4):203-211

[24] Hemalatha RJ, Vijayabaskarin V. Histogram based synovitis scoring system using ultrasound images of rheumatoid arthritis. Journal of Clinical and Diagnostic Research. 2018;**12**(8):LC10-LC14

[25] Niu S, Chen Q, de Sisternes L, Rubin DL, Zhang W, Liu Q. Automated retinal layers segmentation in SD-OCT images using dual-gradient and spatial correlation smoothness constraint. Computers in Biology and Medicine. 2015;**54**:116-128

[26] Guo J, Shi F, Zhu W, Chen H, Chen X. A framework for classification and segmentation of branch retinal artery occlusion in SD-OCT. Prog Biomed Opt Imaging - Proc SPIE. 2016;**9784**(7):3518-3527

[27] Hussain MA, Bhuiyan A, Turpin A, Luu CD, Theodre Smith R, Guymer RH, et al. Automatic identification of pathology-distorted retinal layer boundaries using SD-OCT imaging. IEEE Transactions on Biomedical Engineering. 2017;**64**(7):1638-1649

Chapter 10

A New Method to Manipulate Conventional OCT Images to Measure Changes in the Relative Haemoglobin Oxygen Saturation

Erwin-Michel Davila-Iniesta and Luis Niño-de-Rivera

Abstract

Conventional OCT gray scale images hidden information that do not let the physician to measure the retina oxygen blood saturation. We discuss in this chapter a new approach to extract valuable information from conventional OCT images. The main idea is to convert OCT images to colored images that let the physician to identify more easily the complex structures at the retina circulatory network. A key point in this chapter is not only to identify OCT differences through illness, but also to find a metrics to predict the percent (%) of oxygen saturation in the eye fundus. We will focus on the difficulties to measure oxygen saturation within the ocular vasculature from light reflection. Discussion concerns about a new metric to measure the oxygen saturation within the blood vessels from OCT images. We propose to transmit the lecturer the need to take advantage of the properties within HbO_2 and Hb when absorbing light and how that absorption reflected in gray color intensity can be converted as an algorithm to measure the oxygen saturation numerically.

Keywords: choroidal structure, fundus images, image processing, OCT image, oxygen saturation, preprocessing filters, Pseudocolor method, retinal microvasculature, retinal oximetry

1. Introduction

Optical coherence tomography (OCT) [1–4] is becoming as a new research field to find new data to study the blood oxygenation from said vessels within inner and outer retina. Noninvasive spectrophotometric retinal oximetry has been a target for over five decades ago. Our work and results reported in this chapter are inspired from a previous experiences reported in Ref. [3]. We invite lectures to study previous reports about OCT image processing [3–8] to follow the evolution of noninvasive spectrophotometric retinal oximetry efforts. However, image processing from optical coherence tomography (OCT) requires new alternatives to analyze the absorption difference between oxyhemoglobin (HbO_2) and deoxyhemoglobin (Hb) in the retinal vessels.

OCT images show an internal view of the eye. The inside view of the ocular eye is recorded through the pupil, and this let to get an image that shows the vascular system inside the ocular glove [1]. The study is performed by projecting a beam of light into the pupil to facilitate the visualization of the fundus. Fundus images let to know if patients have different eye condition, like retinal detachment, retinal thrombosis, macular degeneration, diabetic retinopathy and glaucoma. However, diagnostic steel depends on the physician experience and not in a set of new parameters that can be extracted from the OCT image that converted in new data that let to know from image gray levels to measure the oxygen saturation in the retina vein system [3, 5, 7]. The oxygen saturation that is intrinsically in the gray levels of the OCT image depends directly on the frequency that the image is obtained, which comprises a range between 570 and 600 nm [9–13]. This relationship is clearly shown in **Figures 1** and **2. Figure 2** shows the absorption spectrum of Hb and HbO_2 [9 at 532 nm].

We have now new ideas about vascular retina oximetry (VRO). VRO can be understood as the study of oxygen saturation measurement from OCT conventional images if they are processed properly. We defined the VRO approach as a new method to measure the oxyhemoglobin (HbO_2) and deoxyhemoglobin (Hb) from light reflection at different wavelengths. Light reflection from HbO_2 and Hb is the gray light levels seen from the OCT images. These gray levels are not properly recognized by humans; however, OCT image processing techniques, as discussed in this chapter, are excellent tools converting conventional OCT images in new ones according to light reflectance laws. The calculus of percentage of HbO_2 from OCT images is a big challenge. We present in this chapter a new method to evaluate oxygen saturation at the retina vein system.

The Eyeball structure visualized from a fundus image as shown in **Figure 1**. **Figure 1** shows the main central eye arterial just entering at the optic nerve disk. The main artery divides into the central retina artery and ciliary arteries to supply the inner and outer retina at the back of the eye. However, this image, as shown, is far away to give us information about the oxygen consumption in the vein circulatory

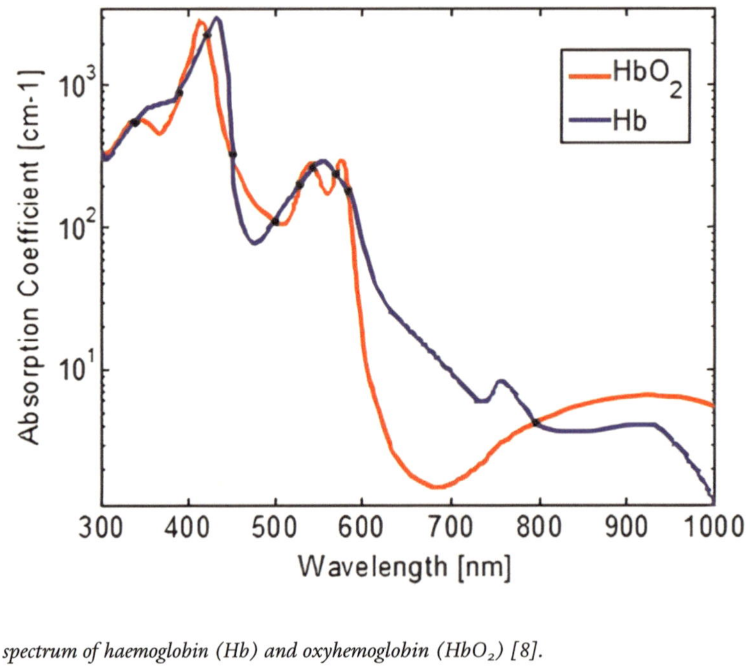

Figure 1.
Absorption spectrum of haemoglobin (Hb) and oxyhemoglobin (HbO_2) [8].

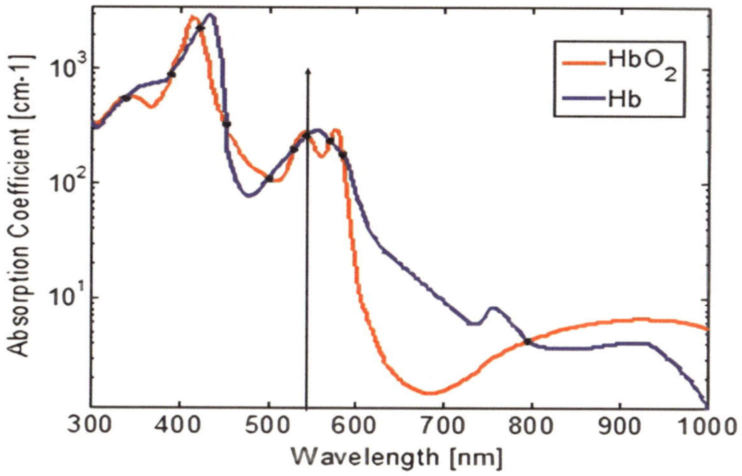

Figure 2.
Plot of the absorption spectrum of Hb and HbO_2 [8], with the absorption spectrum indicator at 532 nm.

system. The human retina is a highly oxygen consuming structure. It happens that the human retina consumes oxygen faster than the brain; consequently, the retina metabolic processes are highly dependent on oxygen saturation $SATO_2$. The choroid has the responsibility to supply oxygen to the cone and rods at the retina complex system.

The transparent structure of the eye fundus offers an extraordinary chance to extract information from the visible vein system about the oxygen going in there. The image spectrometry lets to analyze the oxygen content inside the arterial system if the image is filtered adequately to extract the quantities of oxygen going inside the haemoglobin. This is not an easy task; it is a steel and noncompletely solved problem. The key point is how to measure the absorption of light of haemoglobin and deoxyhemoglobin and from OCT images which vein colors depend on the quantity of oxygen they have in there. The spectral analysis can show both structures as filters that reflect different amounts of light in specific wavelengths depending on its chemical composition; this means more or less oxygen they transport. **Table 1** shows the different wavelengths of the laser bands required to distinguished with higher accuracy between haemoglobin (613 nm) and deoxyhemoglobin (486 nm) [14].

We show in **Figure 3** the relationship between light absorption in Hb and HbO_2 and its relation with the frequency of the light beam. As said above, light absorption and consequently oxygen saturation is a function that depends on the wavelength of the beam light. The optimum frequency to find differences between Hb and HbO_2 are 570 and 600 nm. Jóna Valger›ur Kristjánsdóttir describes important results of light absorption capacity in [9]. Our group and other researchers [3, 5–7, 9, 15] are interested in applying the light

Laser Band	Wavelength (λ)
Red	635*nm*
Green	532*nm*
Blue	486*nm*
Infrared	802*nm*

Table 1.
Table with the different wavelengths of the laser bands [14].

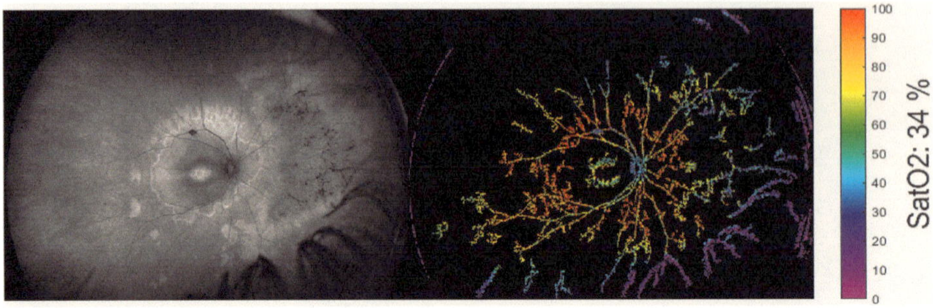

Figure 3.
A. Original fundus image with retinitis pigmentosa obtained at 532nm. B. Image resulting from applying the pseudocolor method to a fundus image with retinitis pigmentosa obtained a 532nm.

absorption blood properties to find differences between Hb and HbO_2 [7]. The main idea goes converting those properties in new colored OCT images where colors let the physician to see the oxygen saturation performance in the retinal vascular system [3].

2. Methodology

The oxygen saturation $SATO_2$ inside the eye circulatory system is highly correlated with the light absorption [16] in each point of the OCT images. Then, the oxygen at the HBO_2 at maximum saturation levels at the corresponding wavelengths shown in **Figure 3** will show the maximum absorbance of light. This absorbance is shown in an OCT image as the light intensity output filtered by the veins. The OCT emitter light or input light to the veins has a specific frequency according to spectral answer as shown in **Figure 3**. Obviously, the Hb has the lower $SATO_2$ since Hb is the blood returning after delivering the oxygen to the retina. Hb will absorb light according to the blue curve as shown in **Figure 3**. It is well known that arterial blood is red and venues blood is blue. This color differences and oxygen saturation can be seen too in a black and white OCT image. Now consider the image in **Figure 1** as a black and white image. Notice that the black and white image shown in **Figure 4** is now the negative version of the black and white image in **Figure 1**. Then, the light reflected from the Hb system will show the less reflected light in comparison with the light reflected by the HBO_2. This means that in the black and white version of **Figure 1**, the highest white illumination will correspond to the highest $SATO_2$, while the darkness points in **Figure 4** will show the points with the lower oxygen saturation $SATO_2$. This difference is clearly observed in the blue and green wavelengths graphs in **Figure 3**. Then, HbO_2 has the highest absorption points and are at 418, 542, 577, and 925 nm. However, the Hb has highest absorption points located at: 430, 550, 758, and 910 nm.

We have a big challenge now. This means to implement computational procedures that let estimating the $SATO_2$ from OCT images. The estimation requires calculating true values of oxygen saturation in the eye circulatory system.

2.1 Oxygen calculus of the blood

The $SATO_2$ in HbO_2 can be calculated as the relationship between HbO_2 and the HbO_2 + Hb [17]. This easy relation will give us the percentage of HbO_2 compared with the whole oxygen in both HbO_2 + Hb as shown in Eq. (1):

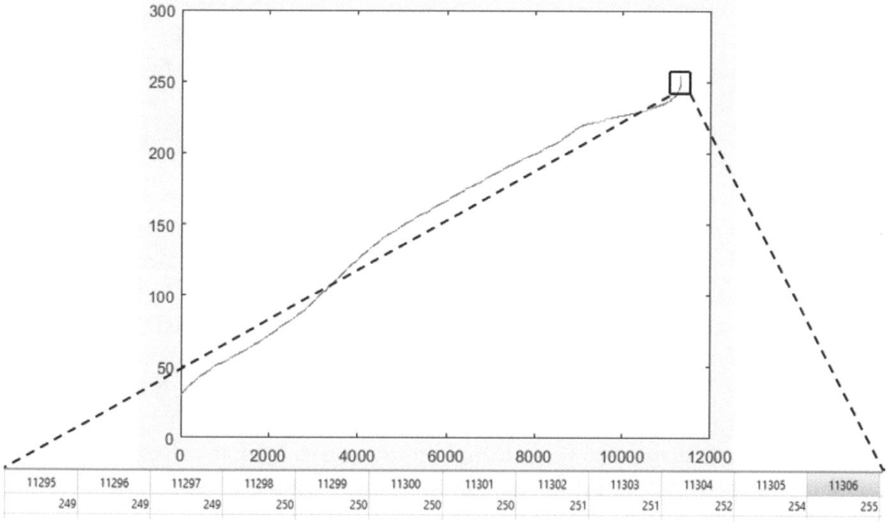

Figure 4.
Plot of grayscale values of ***Figure 3A****.*

$$SatO_2 = \frac{HbO_2}{Hb + HbO_2} \times 100\% \qquad (1)$$

where HbO_2 is the oxygen combined with haemoglobin and Hb is the deoxygenated haemoglobin. The $SatO_2$ is multiplied by 100 to express the $SatO_2$ in percentage. The $SatO_2$ of blood goes to 97,5–75% at 100 mmHg for the mixed venous blood.

OCT black and white images as shown in **Figure 4** are normalized to get a set of levels going from 0 to 255. The 0 represents the highest level of darkness or lowest level of illumination. The 255 levels represent the maximum white intensity. The HbO_2 with the highest $SatO_2$ will be represented with the 255 gray level. Then, we have a new easy way to evaluate the $SatO_2$ in the circulatory ocular globe system (COGS). This new approach considers as a vector only the pixels in the veins shown in the black and white OCT. The veins are filtered by a segmentation algorithm that converts the circulatory eye system as a numerical matrix. This matrix depending on their values between o and 255 let identify the differences in $SatO_2$ in veins and consequently will implement new alternatives to show the physician the performance of the circulatory eye system in normal and illness conditions:

$$SatO_2 = \frac{\sum_{n=96}^{N-1} \frac{P_{n_{total}}}{255}}{\sum_{n=1}^{N-1} \frac{P_k}{95} + \sum_{n=96}^{N-1} \frac{P_{n_{total}}}{255}} \times 100\% \qquad (2)$$

where $P_{n_{total}}$ is

$$P_{n_{total}} = \sum_{n=96}^{N-1} \frac{P_{n_1}}{199} + \sum_{n=200}^{N-1} \frac{P_{n_2}}{255} \qquad (3)$$

Eq. 2 let calculate $SATO_2$ from an OCT gray levels image analogously as Eq. (1) does. The OCT image converted as a vector is a matrix, where each number in there represents the proportion of light absorbance by HBO_2; consequently, it is a measure of the oxygen in an specific pixel depending on its value, the 255 value, and the highest gray level has the highest oxygen absorption in that pixel and so on for lower values in the 1 to 255 gray levels scale.

P_k in Eq. (2) is the value of the vector in pixel k. In Eq. 2, we consider that the vector P_k belonging to venous blood pixels going from 1 to 95.

$P_{n\ total}$ in eq. (3) with two variables P_{n_1} and P_{n_2} are the pixel values of each vector to be analyzed. In this case, P_{n_1} takes the values that are delimited by the n and the dividend, and these values will vary between 96 and 199, which are the values proposed in this work for the representation of venous haemoglobin. On the other hand, P_{n_2} will take the values from 200 to 255 which are the values proposed to identify the arterial haemoglobin or oxyhemoglobin. Thus, when the substitution of the variables is made, the result is $P_{n_{total}}$ which is the whole amount of gray levels in the vector. This includes all the pixels representing the arterial and venous system. The arterial and venous systems are normalized to their maximum values. Hb has values from 1 to 95, HbO_2 venous goes from 96 to 199, and HbO_2 arterial goes from 200 to 255.

We finally arrive to a final $SatO_2$ equation as shown below:

$$SatO_2 = \frac{\sum_{n=96}^{N-1} \frac{P_{n_1}}{199} + \sum_{n=200}^{N-1} \frac{P_{n_2}}{255}}{\sum_{n=1}^{N-1} \frac{P_k}{95} + \left(\sum_{n=96}^{N-1} \frac{P_{n_1}}{199} + \sum_{n=200}^{N-1} \frac{P_{n_2}}{255}\right)} \times 100\% \tag{4}$$

As a matter of fact of Eq. 4 with the following values, $P_{n_1} = 138$, $P_{n_2} = 225$, and $P_k = 80$shows $SAtO_2$ calculation for pixel in $k = 80$:

$$SatO_2 = \frac{138/199 + 225/255}{80/95 + (138/199 + 225/255)} \times 100\% \tag{5}$$

$$SatO_2 = \frac{1.5758}{2.4179} \times 100\% \tag{6}$$

$$SatO_2 = 0.6517 \times 100\% = 65.17\% \tag{7}$$

Then in (7), 65.17% is the $SATO_2$ for pixel in $k = 80$.

The assignment of colors to the different gray level values was as follows: 0–black, 1–32 equals purple, 33–64 violet, 65–95 blue, 96–127 cyan, 128–159 green, 160–191 yellow, 192–223 orange, and 224–255 red. Then Eq. (3) can evaluate $SatO_2$ by regions or specific borders inside the OCT image.

We can see from the above discussion that we have a new numerical method to calculate $SatO_2$. This calculus let describes all the pixels at the circulatory eye system as numbers that represents each one the $SatO_2$ by pixel. The $SatO_2$ can be expressed too as a color vein map for an easy recognition of the physician about the state of the circulatory system and its relation with oxygen performance.

3. Results

Figure 3 shows the result of applying the pseudocolor method to an image that was obtained at 532*nm* with the OPTOS California retinograph (this retinograph works with different wavelengths as shown in **Table 1**), according to gray levels shown in **Figure 4**.

Notice that in **Figure 2** at 532 nm, there is no difference between the absorption spectrum of Hb and HbO_2. However, our results show that differences in gray levels (128–255) let find $SatO_2$ differences, shown as red and green $SatO_2$ levels in **Figure 3**. This is due to the good pseudocolor sensitivity segmentation method discussed above. The same can be said with the red and blue (HbO_2 and Hb) intersections points in **Figure 2**.

We find in **Figure 4** the OCT image vector shown as the blue curve. The blue vector has seven changes we recognize as slopes, and each slope was associated with the $SatO_2$ variation in a specific region of set of gray levels [18] according to the absorbance properties of Hb and HbO_2, as shown in **Figure 2**.

We show in **Figures 5–8** the $SatO_2$ absorbance results from images obtained with wavelengths: 486*nm*, 635*nm*, 802*nm*, and the combination of the wavelengths 532*nm* and 635*nm*.

We show in **Figures 5–8** the results obtained with the pseudocolor method. Color levels show differences in $SatO_2$ in the ocular microvasculature system. This method as shown can be applied to both fundus images and angiographies. It is important to say that **Figure 8** shows the $SatO_2$ of the choroid, making a novel method to analyze the vasculature of the choroid from the vector obtained by the pseudocolor method.

The pseudocolor method allows to differentiate clearly the microvasculature of the fundus and then to analyze the vasculature performance from new tools.

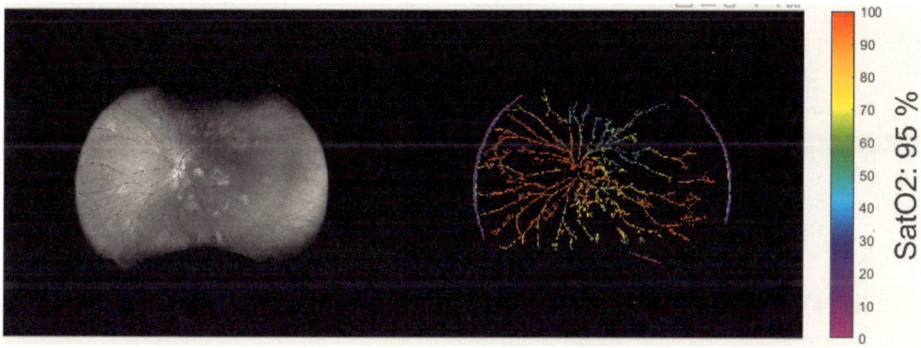

Figure 5.
A. Original healthy fundus image obtained at 635nm. B. Image resulting from applying the pseudocolor method to a healthy fundus image obtained at 635nm.

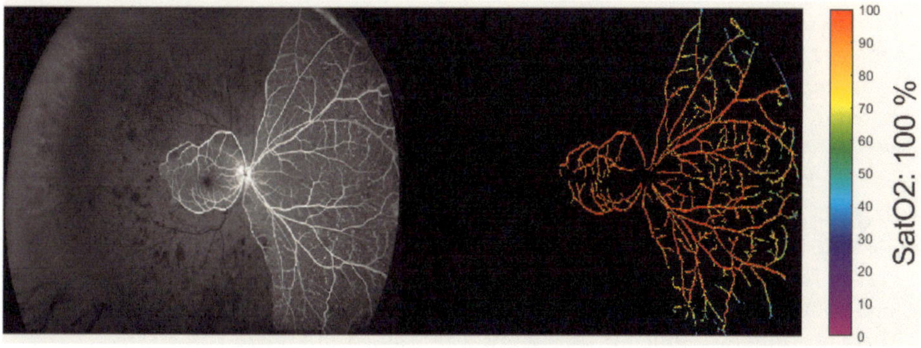

Figure 6.
A. Original ocular fundus image with ocular ischemia obtained at 486nm. B. Image resulting from applying the pseudocolor method to a fundus image with ocular ischemia obtained a 486nm.

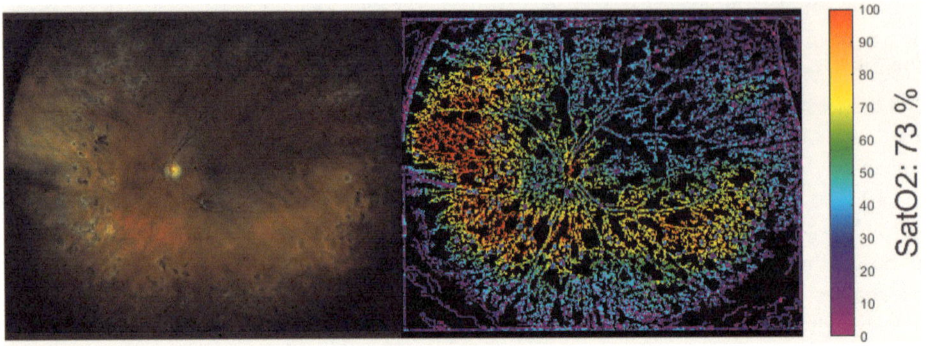

Figure 7.
A. Original fundus image with retinitis pigmentosa with the combination of wavelengths. 532nm and 635nm. B. Image resulting from applying the pseudocolor method to a fundus image with the combination of wavelengths. 532nm and 635nm.

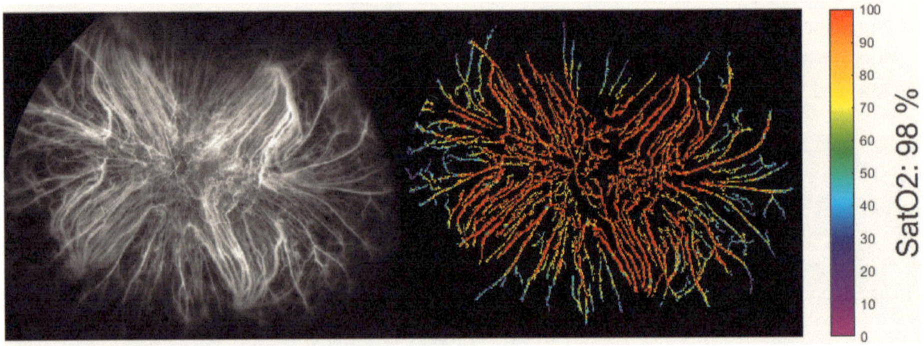

Figure 8.
A. Original fundus image of the choroid obtained with a wavelength of 802nm. B. Image resulting from applying the pseudocolor method to a fundus image of the choroid obtained with a wavelength at 802nm.

We show in **Figure 9A**, with author permission, the $SatO_2$ reported by Kristjánsdóttir et al. [4]. As a matter of comparison, we show the same image obtained at 570 nm (**Figure 9B**) and 600 nm (**Figure 9C**) applying our method with results shown in **Figures 10** and **11**.

The resulting images in **Figures 10** and **11** obtained with the method presented in this chapter show notable differences in the color assignment among Kristjánsdóttir et al. and ours; as mentioned in the methodology, the oxygen saturation formula proposed in here was applied in this assignment, and this explains the difference between results reported in [4] and ours; however, color standardization requires deeper work. It is clear that wavelength has an important role to find best results when looking HbO_2 or Hb. **Figure 11** shows results with 570 nm image, and **Figure 10** shows results with 600 nm.

Figure 12A–C shows results published by Geirsdottir et al. [3], which is similar to the one obtained by Kristjánsdóttir et al. [4].

The algorithm developed in this work was applied in **Figure 12A** to see how our method compares with Geirsdottir et al. and our results are shown in **Figure 13**.

We show in **Figure 14** the pseudocolor method applied in the original **Figure 12B**.

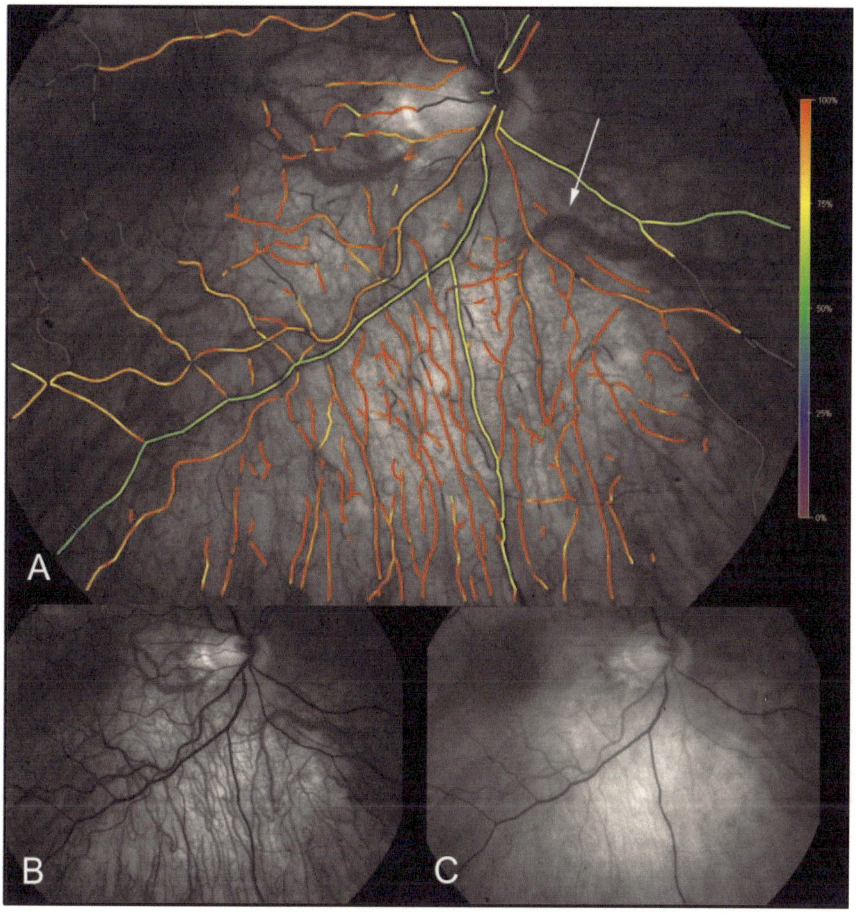

Figure 9.
*Oximetry of the eye obtained at 570 nm (**Figure 9B**), and 600 nm (**Figure 9C**).*

The first results obtained by Davila-Iniesta et al. [3] will be compared with the pseudocolor method as shown in **Figures 15–18**. We find an improvement in the segmentation procedure. We find that pseudocolor method provides a better

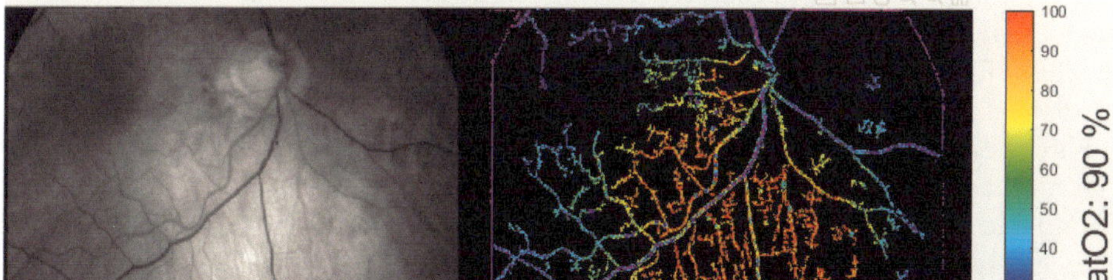

Figure 10.
*False color method applied to **Figure 9C**.*

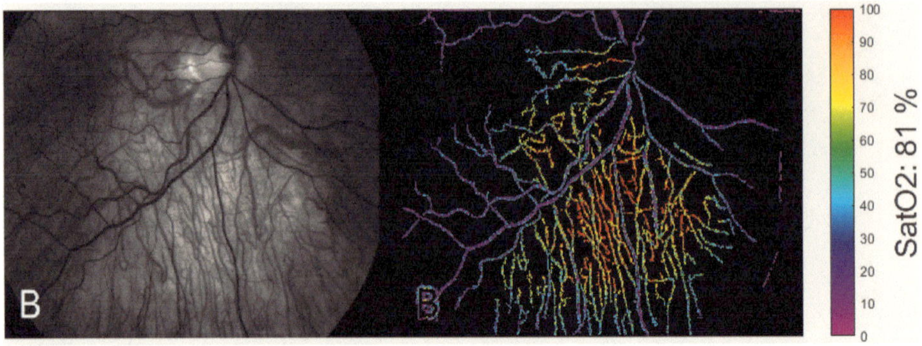

Figure 11.
False color method applied to ***Figure 9B****.*

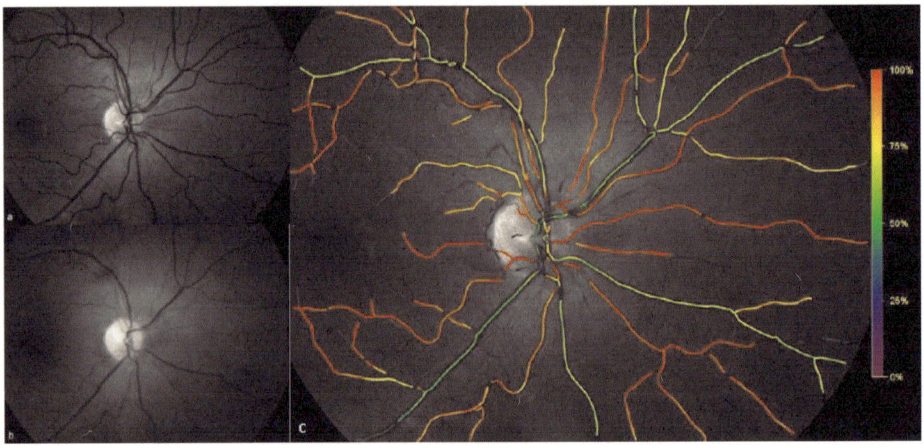

Figure 12.
*Eye oximetry obtained at 570 nm (****Figure 12A****), and 600 nm (****Figure 12B****).*

resolution with vein network and gives a whole scheme about the distribution of the $SatO_2$ at the vein system.

Figure 16B shows a healthy eye, and using the pseudocolor proposed method we noticed an improvement in the vein network sight in relation to the original fundus image [3, 4]. We show too that it is possible to see the $SatO_2$ levels converted as a color set. This will help the physician to a better understanding of the performance of the vasculature system.

Figure 17A shows the fundus image with macular edema. After applying the false color method, the resulting image shown in **Figure 17B** was obtained. We find that the relationship between macular edema and $SatO_2$ plays an important role. However, this statement requires statistical analysis from enough of this illness OCT images, and statically analysis can be applied since we have converted every images in a numerical vector.

Figure 18B shows the fundus image with macular edema after applying the pseudocolor method. The $SatO_2$ ratio in this image is seen to be clearer than the previous image. Also, the microvascular system and how it is affected due to this disease can be seen.

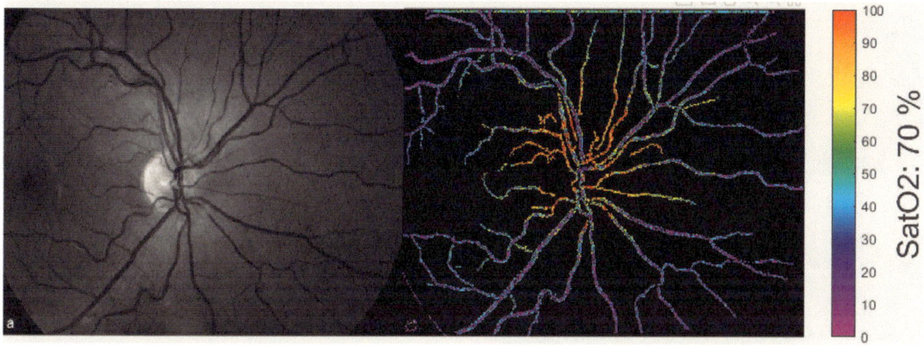

Figure 13.
*Pseudocolor method applied to **Figure 12A**.*

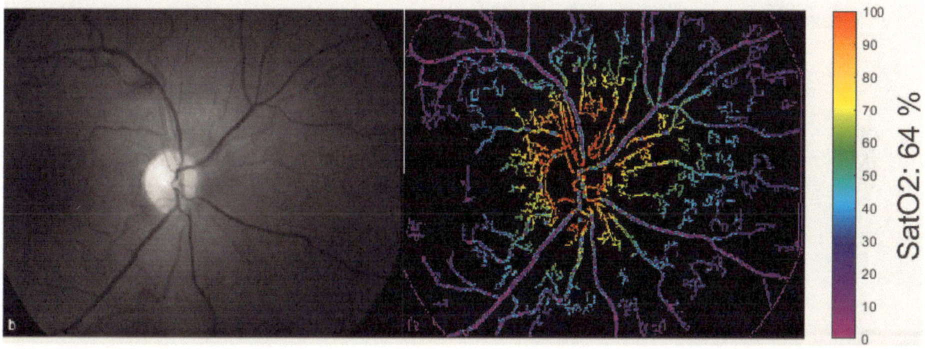

Figure 14.
*False color method applied to **Figure 12B**.*

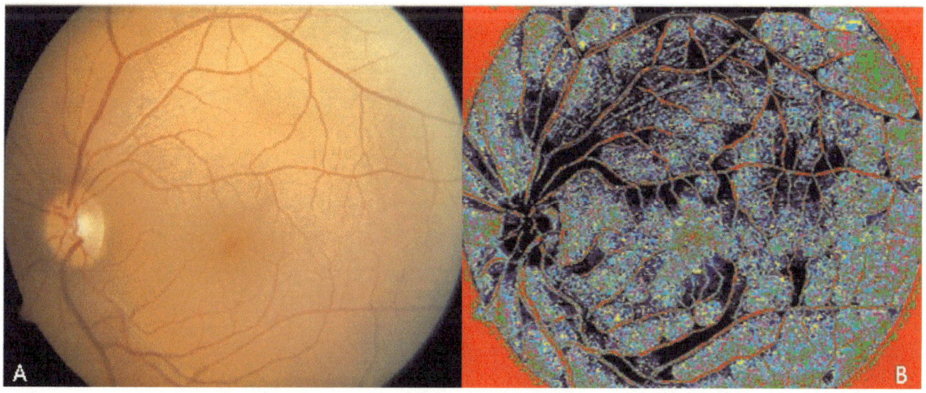

Figure 15.
A. Fundus image of healthy eye. B. False color method applied to the fundus image [3].

We show in **Table 2** how the eye circulatory system transformed as vector can be analyzed from excel tools an even by more advanced ones like Jupiter Notebook tools.

We show in **Figure 19** an important result. The vector means that the OCT image at different frequencies is now represented as a distribution function. We find at the X

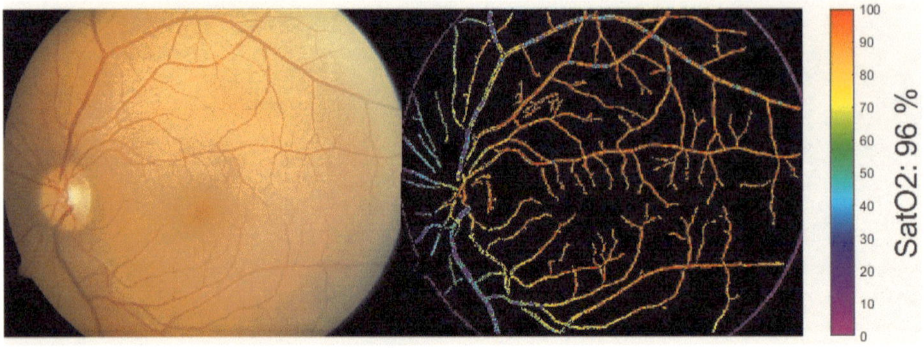

Figure 16.
*A. Fundus image of healthy eye. B. Pseudocolor method applied to **Figure 15A**.*

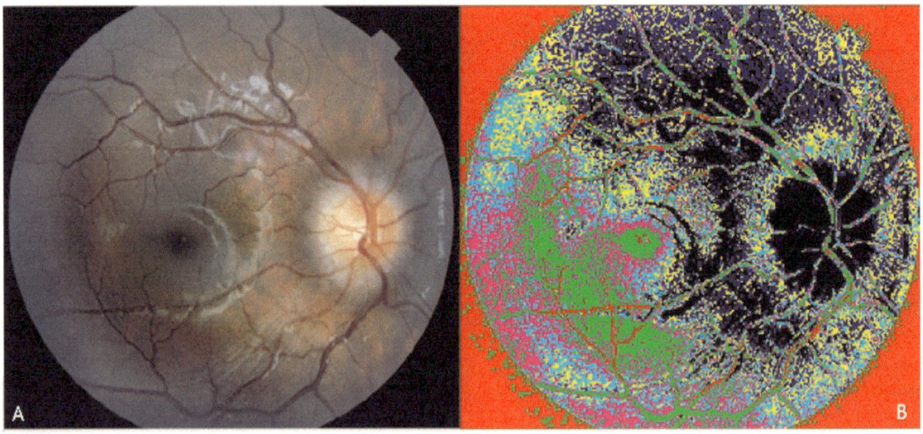

Figure 17.
*A. Fundus image with macular edema. B. False color method applied to **Figure 17A**.*

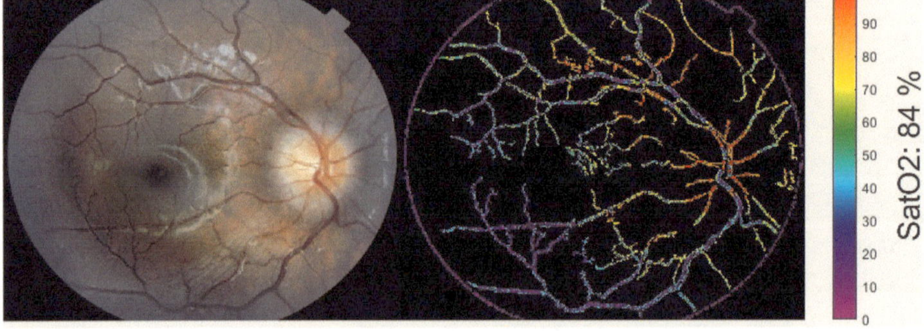

Figure 18.
*A. Fundus image with macular edema. B. Pseudocolor method applied to **Figure 17A**.*

axis the 0 to 255 gray levels and at the Y axis the count of pixels belonging to that level. This new representation of $SatO_2$ gives an exact picture about the performance of the vein eye system. Taking a look at **Figure 19** Healthy eye-1, we notice clearly the distribution of $SatO_2$ in the fondues vein system. The maximum $SatO_2$ values are in

Choroid (802 nm) – vector	Choroid (802 nm) – pur& $$$;	Choroid (802 nm) – Gr& $$$;	Choroid (802 nm) – Bl& $$$;	Choroid (802 nm) – Cy& $$$;	Choroid (802 nm) – Gre& $$$;	Choroid (802 nm) – Yellow&$$$;	Choroid (802 nm) – Ora& $$$;	Choroid (802 nm) – &$ $$;
31	31	34	65	96	128	160	192	224
32	32	34	65	96	128	160	192	224
34		35	65	96	128	160	192	224
34		36	65	96	128	160	192	224
35		37	65	96	128	160	192	224
36		37	65	96	128	160	192	224
37		37	65	96	128	160	192	224
37		38	65	96	128	160	192	224
37		38	65	96	128	160	192	224
38		39	65	96	128	160	192	224
38		39	65	96	128	160	192	224
39		40	65	96	128	160	192	224
39		40	65	96	128	160	192	224
40		40	65	96	128	160	192	224
40		41	65	96	128	160	192	224
40		42	65	96	128	160	192	224
41		42	65	96	128	160	192	224
42		42	65	96	128	160	192	224
42		43	65	96	128	160	192	224

Table 2.
Shows only 20 rows from 40,302 of the real data set for an OCT image.

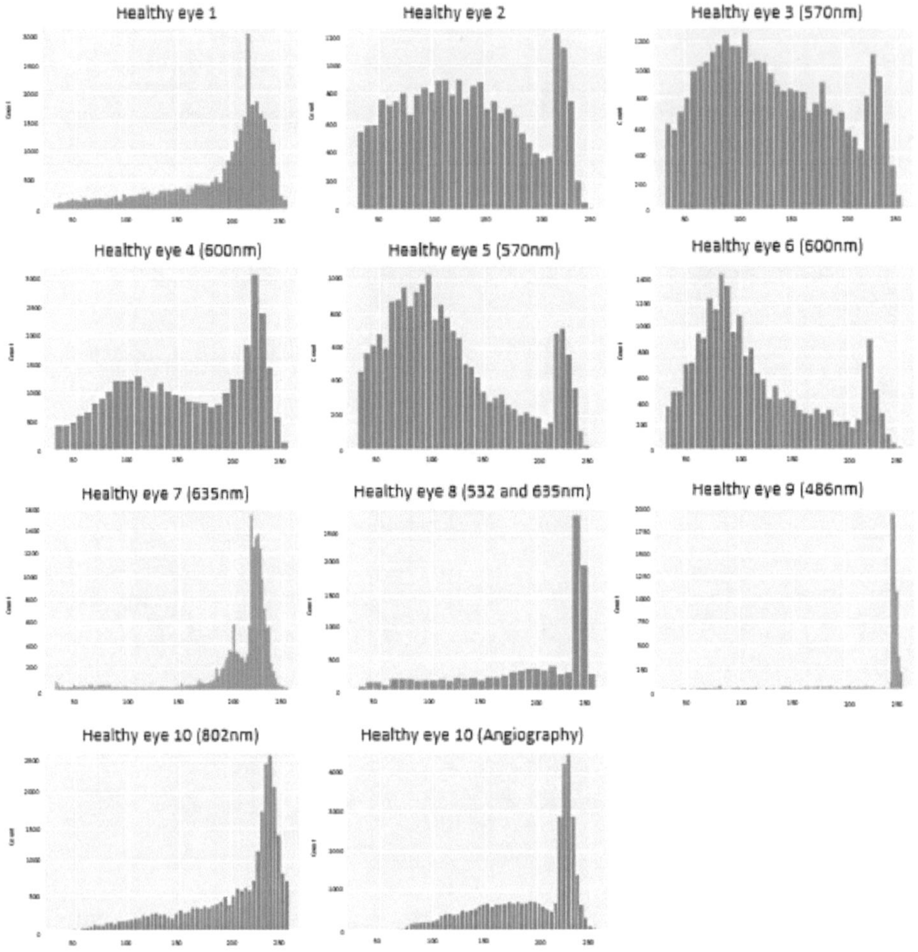

Figure 19.
Histogram of different OCT images. Horizontal axis represent the 0 to 255 gray levels and vertical axis represent the count per level.

the range between 190 and 240 gray levels, just inside the HBO_2. The lowest $SatO_2$ levels are between 0 and 95 gray levels, belonging to the HB. **Figure 19** shows that we can find a set of clearly different $SatO_2$ distributions, and this is an important result since we can find detailed differences numerically represented that cannot be distinguished by traditional human visual OCT analysis. This of course is not a conclusive statement; however, first results go to that direction.

4. Discussion

We discussed in this chapter a new way to observe OCT images and angiographies. Observing the eye circulatory veins colored analogous to $SATO_2$, we give physician and researches new alternatives to look at the inner eye blood system from a numerical perspective. This will let to follow up to people suffering from various diseases not only from the clinic perspective but also from the statistical performance that affects the oxygen saturation of an eye.

DOI: http://dx.doi.org/10.5772/intechopen.110884

It is the case of a statistical analysis which allows to see how the behavior of the vector of the image is being analyzed, as well as, to separate the values that are believed to be within the curve as shown in **Figure 4** and to give guidelines for future research in this area.

This new method to manipulate conventional OCT images to measure changes in the relative haemoglobin oxygen saturation let the physician to know the $SatO_2$ as a set of numerical data, and then the physician will know the $SatO_2$ at each point of the circulatory system. The fact that the OCT image is transformed into a matrix where each pixel of the circulatory eye system has a specific gray level and then a corresponding $SatO_2$ measurement will let to follow up the performance of oxygen saturation through each branch of the circulatory system. As said above, we have the $SatO_2$ as a set of gray levels perfectly defined into 0 to 255. We showed in our results (**Figures 19** and **20**) a new way to look at the choroid in **Figure 8**, and notice that this new representation gives a bar plot measuring how the oxygen saturation is changing through sets of colors (gray levels). This procedure will let study the patient evolution by comparing the performance of bar plots through time.

The effects of $SatO_2$ in degenerative eye illness like glaucoma, RP, and diabetes among others can be studied statistically following the changes in the $SatO_2$ distribution function, comparing a big set of variables involved in the diseases, finding possible correlation among many variables, for instance, between blood sugar levels and its effects in $SatO_2$ choroids.

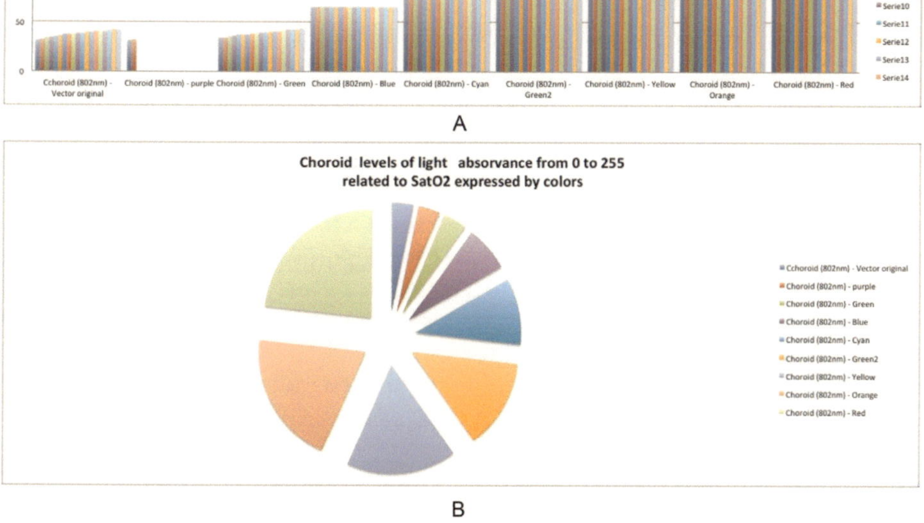

Figure 20.
A. Choroid levels of light absorbance. B. Shows the distribution of SatO2 from nine different levels of SatO2 concentration presented as color from 0 to 255.

Our method for measuring oxygen saturation in the eye using OCT imaging represents a significant improvement over current methods in terms of accuracy and traceability. While conventional methods use an average measurement of oxygen saturation in the eye, our method provides a detailed map of oxygen saturation throughout the ocular circulation. This may have significant implications for the diagnosis and monitoring of ocular diseases related to oxygen saturation, such as retinal vascular disease. In addition, our method is based on existing OCT images, making it more accessible and less expensive than invasive and advanced imaging methods currently used in the clinic. Overall, we believe that our work can significantly contribute to the understanding of ocular physiology and improve eye care in the future.

This approach opens great opportunities to make big data OCT sets that can be evaluated even by artificial intelligence and machine learning tools.

5. Conclusions and future challenges

Authors propose a new mathematical expression that allows the calculation of oxygen saturation from conventional OCT images in a computational way. The new results discussed in this chapter shows that pseudocolor method gives better results now than those previously reported in our paper "False Color Method for Retinal Oximetry" [3]. The results obtained need deeper validation by assigning colors to the gray scale depending on the OCT manufacturer. Then for a specific OCT at the same frequency, all gray levels 0 to 255 will be the same trough any study, and then we have the same reference, which means comparison among images from the same OCT is valid. OCT operation frequency plays a significant role in gray levels distribution, as shown in **Figure 19**. This means that for a specific clinic study for illness or patients follow-up, we recommend to use the same equipment and frequency in order to have the same reference through the study. Traditional OCT visual analysis does not let making difference for each of the 0 to 255 gray level in a OCT image. However, it is clear that the $SatO_2$ distribution function let us know clearly how the $SatO_2$ distribution is changing, but we must be careful about different OCT frequencies at time to take the OCT image. Different OCT frequency gives important changes in the OCT gray-level image distribution. This is well known from the spectrographic performance of HBO and HBO_2 at different light wavelengths; fortunately, we have now numerically documented those differences with the distribution function of the gray levels of OCT at different frequencies as shown in results (see **Figure 19**).

In future work, we require some preprocessing OCT images to improve the results obtained by the proposed $SatO_2$ procedures. New opportunities are coming from the statistical study of the color levels assigned to the image and thus the evolution of gray levels through illness. The OCT images converted as vectors open new opportunities to study the complex structure of the retina from the $SatO_2$ effects. Then, this new tool provides a numerical approach for a better understanding of degenerative eye illness.

Acknowledgements

The authors thank CONACyT and Instituto Politecnico Nacional for their financial support throughout the work.

DOI: http://dx.doi.org/10.5772/intechopen.110884

Conflict of interest

The authors declare that they have no conflicts of interest.

Author details

Erwin-Michel Davila-Iniesta and Luis Niño-de-Rivera*
Artificial Vision Lab, ESIME UC, Instituto Politécnico Nacional, IPN México, México

*Address all correspondence to: luisninoderivera@gmail.com

References

[1] Graue-Wiechers E, Graue-Hernandez E. Ophthalmology in the Practice of General Medicine. 3rd ed. Mexico: McGraw Hill; 2009

[2] Saceda-Corralo D. Fundus Examination. 2019. Available from: https://www.webconsultas.com/pruebas-medicas/examen-de-fondo-de-ojo-11462

[3] Davila-Iniesta E, Guerrero-Gonzalez S, Santiago-Amaya J, Castillo-Juarez P, Niño de Rivera-Oyarzabal L. False color method for retinal oximetry. Journal of Biomedical Science and Engineering. 2019;**12**:533-544

[4] MATLAB. Image Thresholding. de MATLAB Sitio web: Available from: https://la.mathworks.com/discovery/image-thresholding.html

[5] Geirsdottir A, Palsson O, Hardarson SH, Olafsdottir OB, Kristjansdottir JV, Stefánsson E. Retinal vessel oxygen saturation in healthy individuals. Investigative Ophthalmology & Visual Science. 2012;**53**(9):5433-5442

[6] Kristjansdottir JV, Hardarson SH, Harvey AR, Olafsdottir OB, Eliasdottir TS, Stefánsson E. Choroidal oximetry with a noninvasive spectrophotometric oximeter. Investigative Ophthalmology & Visual Science. 2013;**54**(5):3234-3239

[7] Palsson O, Geirsdottir A, Hardarson SH, Olafsdottir OB, Kristjansdottir JV, Stefánsson E. Retinal oximetry images must Be standardized: A methodological analysis. Investigative Ophthalmology & Visual Science. 2012;**53**(4):1729-1733

[8] Liu H, Ivanov K, Wang Y, Wang L. A novel method based on two cameras for accurate estimation of arterial oxygen saturation. Biomedical Engineering Online. 2015;**14**:3

[9] Not Without My Glasses. Visual Health in Mexico: half population needs glasses. 2018. Available from: http://www.nosinmisgafas.info/blog/salud-visual/salud-visual-mexico

[10] Olafsdottir OB, Vandewalle E, Abegao-Pinto L, Geirsdottir A, de Clerck E, Stalmans P, et al. Retinal oxygen metabolism in healthy subjects and glaucoma patients. The British Journal of Ophthalmology. 2014;**98**(3):329-333

[11] Eliasdottir TS, Bragason D, Hardarson SH, Vacchiano C, Gislason T, Valgerdur-Kristjansdottir J, et al. Retinal oximetry measures systemic hipoxia in central nervous system vessels in chronic obstructive pulmonary disease. PLoS One. 2017;**12**(3):e0174026

[12] Paul JP, O'Connel RA, Hosking SL, Anderson AJ, Bui BV. Retinal oxygen saturation: Novel analysis method for the Oxymap. Optometry and Vision Science. 2013;**90**(10):1104-1110. DOI: 10.1097/opx.0000000000000028

[13] Hardarson SH, Harris A, Karlsson RA, Halldorsson GH, Kagemann L, Rechtman E, et al. Automatic retinal oximetry. Investigative Ophthalmology & Visual Science. 2006;**47**(11):5011-5016. DOI: 10.1167/iovs.06-0039

[14] OPTOS. California icg was developed for retinal specialists to optimize management of AMD, uveitic conditions and other choroidal pathology. 2018. Available from: https://www.optos.com/en/products/california-icg/

[15] Orthopedics Online. What is a pulse oximeter, how does it work and why is it key in the fight against COVID-19. 2021. Available from: Orthopedics MIMAS

Website: https://www.ortopediamimas.com/blog-de-ortopedia/que-es-un-pulsioximetro-como-funciona-y-por-que-es-clave-en-la-lucha-contra-la-covid-19/

[16] Chan ED, Chan MM, Chan MM. Pulse oximetry: Understanding its basic principles facilitates appreciation of its limitations. Respiratory Medicine. 2013; **107**(6):789-799. DOI: 10.1016/j.rmed.2013.02.004

[17] Understanding Pulse Oxymetry SpO2 Concepts. (s/f). Philips.com. 2003. Sitio web: Available from: https://www.documents.philips.com/doclib/enc/fetch/586262/586457/Understanding_Pulse_Oximetry.pdf

[18] UV. Pseudocolor y Falso color. de UV Sitio web: Available from: https://www.uv.es/gpoei/eng/Pfc_web/generalidades/pseudocolor/pseudocolor.htm